STUDY GUIDE TO
PREVENTIVE MEDICAL CARE IN PSYCHIATRY

A Case Approach

STUDY GUIDE TO
PREVENTIVE MEDICAL CARE IN PSYCHIATRY

A Case Approach

Edited by

Robert M. McCarron, D.O.

Glen L. Xiong, M.D.

Craig R. Keenan, M.D.

Lorin M. Scher, M.D.

Jaesu Han, M.D.

Mark E. Servis, M.D.

AMERICAN
PSYCHIATRIC
ASSOCIATION
PUBLISHING

Manufactured in the United States of America on acid-free paper
20 19 18 17 16 5 4 3 2 1
First Edition

American Psychiatric Association Publishing
1000 Wilson Boulevard
Arlington, VA 22209-3901
www.appi.org

Contents

SECTION II

Cardiovascular and Pulmonary Disorders in the Psychiatric Patient Population

Section Editor: Glen L. Xiong, M.D.

Matthew Reed, M.D., M.S.P.H.

Sara Teasdale, M.D., and Christine Kho, M.D.

SECTION III

Endocrine and Metabolic Disorders in the Psychiatric Patient Population

Section Editor: Craig R. Keenan, M.D.

Lindsey Enoch, M.D.

Julie Hylton, M.D., and Stephany Sanchez, M.D.

SECTION IV

Infectious Disorders in the Psychiatric Patient Population

Section Editor: Craig R. Keenan, M.D.

Chinonyerem J. Okwara, M.D.

George K. Gallardo, M.D., and Heather A. Vierra, M.D.

SECTION V

Oncological Disorders in the Psychiatric Patient Population

Section Editors: Jaesu Han, M.D., and Lorin M. Scher, M.D.

Amy Nuismer, M.D.

Katerina Christiansen, M.D.

SECTION VI

Geriatric Preventive Care

Section Editors: Jaesu Han, M.D., and Lorin M. Scher, M.D.

Erica Heiman, M.D.

Aleea Maye, M.D., and Steven R. Chan, M.D. M.B.A.

SECTION VII

Child and Adolescent Preventive Care

Section Editor: Glen L. Xiong, M.D.

Matthew Gibson, M.D.

Danielle Alexander, M.D.

SECTION VIII

Pain Medicine in the Psychiatric Patient Population

Section Editor: Robert M. McCarron, D.O., DFAPA

Kristian Delgado, M.D.

Naileshni Singh, M.D., Amir Ramezani, Ph.D., and Matthew Reed, M.D., M.S.P.H.

PART 2
ANSWER GUIDE

Contributors

Danielle Alexander, M.D.
Combined Family Medicine/Psychiatry Resident Physician, Department of Psychiatry and Behavioral Sciences and Department of Family and Community Medicine, University of California, Davis, School of Medicine, Sacramento, California

Steven R. Chan, M.D., M.B.A.
Senior Resident Physician, Department of Psychiatry and Behavioral Sciences, University of California, Davis, School of Medicine, Sacramento, California

Katerina Christiansen, M.D.
Resident Physician, Department of Internal Medicine, University of California, Davis, Health System, Sacramento, California

Kristian Delgado, M.D.
Advanced Pain Care Clinic, Woodway, Texas

Jeremy DeMartini, M.D.
Combined Internal Medicine/Psychiatry Resident Physician, Department of Internal Medicine and Department of Psychiatry and Behavioral Sciences, University of California, Davis, School of Medicine, Sacramento, California

Lindsey Enoch, M.D.
Chief Resident, Combined Internal Medicine/Psychiatry Resident Physician, Department of Internal Medicine and Department of Psychiatry and Behavioral Sciences, University of California, Davis, School of Medicine, Sacramento, California

George K. Gallardo, M.D.
Internal Medicine Resident Physician, Department of Internal Medicine, University of California, Davis, School of Medicine, Sacramento, California

Matthew Gibson, M.D.
Combined Family Medicine/Psychiatry Resident Physician, Department of Psychiatry and Behavioral Sciences and Department of Family and Community Medicine, University of California, Davis, School of Medicine, Sacramento, California

Jaesu Han, M.D.
Associate Clinical Professor, Department of Psychiatry and Behavioral Sciences, University of California, Davis, School of Medicine, Sacramento, California

Erica Heiman, M.D.
Resident Physician, Department of Internal Medicine, University of California, Davis, School of Medicine, Sacramento, California

Julie Hylton, M.D.
Resident Physician, Department of Psychiatry and Behavioral Sciences, University of California, Davis, School of Medicine, Sacramento, California

Craig R. Keenan, M.D.
Professor and Director, Internal Medicine Residency Program, Department of Internal Medicine of Medicine, University of California, Davis, School of Medicine, Sacramento, California

Christine Kho, M.D.
Combined Internal Medicine/Psychiatry Resident Physician, Department of Internal Medicine and Department of Psychiatry and Behavioral Sciences, University of California, Davis, School of Medicine, Sacramento, California

David Liu, M.D., M.S.
Health Sciences Assistant Clinical Professor, Psychosomatic Medicine Service, Department of Psychiatry and Behavioral Sciences, University of California, Davis, School of Medicine, Sacramento, California

Aleea Maye, M.D.
Combined Internal Medicine/Psychiatry Resident Physician, Department of Internal Medicine and Department of Psychiatry and Behavioral Sciences, University of California, Davis, School of Medicine, Sacramento, California

Robert M. McCarron, D.O., DFAPA
Associate Professor; Director, Pain Psychiatry and Behavioral Sciences; Director, Internal Medicine/Psychiatry Residency; Co-director, Train New Trainers Primary Care Psychiatry Fellowship, Departments of Psychiatry and Behavioral Sciences, Internal Medicine, and Anesthesiology and Pain Medicine, University of California, Davis, School of Medicine, Sacramento, California

Amy Nuismer, M.D.
Combined Family Medicine/Psychiatry Resident Physician, Department of Psychiatry and Behavioral Sciences and Department of Family and Community Medicine, University of California, Davis, School of Medicine, Sacramento, California

Chinonyerem J. Okwara, M.D.
Combined Internal Medicine/Psychiatry Resident Physician, Department of Internal Medicine and Department of Psychiatry and Behavioral Sciences, University of California, Davis, School of Medicine, Sacramento, California

Amir Ramezani, Ph.D.
Assistant Professor and Associate Director of Behavioral Pain Medicine and Director of Neuropsychology, University of California, Davis, School of Medicine, Sacramento, California

Matthew Reed, M.D., M.S.P.H.
Pain Medicine Fellow, Department of Anesthesiology and Pain Medicine, University of California, Davis, School of Medicine, Sacramento, California

Stephany Sanchez, M.D.
Associate Physician, Department of Internal Medicine, University of California, Davis, School of Medicine, Sacramento, California

Lorin M. Scher, M.D.
Director, Emergency Psychiatry, Psychosomatic Medicine Service; Health Sciences Assistant Clinical Professor, Department of Psychiatry and Behavioral Sciences, University of California, Davis, School of Medicine, Sacramento, California

Mark E. Servis, M.D.
Professor, Department of Psychiatry and Behavioral Sciences; Senior Associate Dean for Medical Education, University of California, Davis, School of Medicine, Sacramento, California

Naileshni Singh, M.D.
Assistant Professor and Director, Education, Division of Pain Medicine and Department of Anesthesiology, University of California, Davis, School of Medicine, Sacramento, California

Sara Teasdale, M.D.
Associate Physician, Department of Internal Medicine, University of California, Davis, School of Medicine, Sacramento, California

Heather A. Vierra, M.D.
Department of Internal Medicine, University of California, Davis, School of Medicine, Sacramento, California

Glen L. Xiong, M.D.
Associate Clinical Professor, Department of Psychiatry and Behavioral Sciences, University of California, Davis, School of Medicine, Sacramento, California

Angie Mung Yan Yu, M.D.
Chief Resident, Combined Internal Medicine/Psychiatry Resident Physician, Department of Internal Medicine and Department of Psychiatry and Behavioral Sciences, University of California, Davis, School of Medicine, Sacramento, California

The volume editors and contributors to this book have no competing interests to report.

Preface

The *Study Guide to Preventive Medical Care in Psychiatry: A Case Approach* is a supplementary text intended to help readers synthesize and understand material in the source book. This volume does not offer outlines or additional figures and is not meant to be used as a stand-alone text. Rather, the study guide highlights the most important topics with practice questions that are not available in the source book.

Each chapter of this study guide corresponds to the chapter of the same number in *Preventive Medical Care in Psychiatry: A Practical Guide for Clinicians,* allowing readers to test their knowledge as they work through the source book. After each question, readers will find thorough explanations supported by references to pages and figures in the source book.

In encountering these clinical vignettes, the reader should gain a greater understanding of preventive medicine in psychiatric care. The questions are designed to illustrate patient management, common comorbidities to psychiatric illness, and treatment guidelines. Addressing medical illnesses often leads to an enhanced quality of life that facilitates better psychiatric care. As health reform continues to move toward models of integrated medical and mental care, it is increasingly important that mental health clinicians learn to combine medical and psychiatric approaches. The purpose of this study guide is to equip mental health clinicians and trainees with the foundations to adapt to this new era in health care.

Dedication

The editors are grateful for the opportunity to learn from those whom we teach and mentor.

Acknowledgments

The editors are most grateful to Mehrbanoo Lashai, M.D., and Kelsey Wong for their dedication as assistant editors of this study guide.

PART 1

STUDY QUESTIONS

SECTION I

Preventive Medical Care in Psychiatry: General Principles

Section Editor:
Robert M. McCarron, D.O., DFAPA

Jeremy DeMartini, M.D.
With
Angie Mung Yan Yu, M.D.
David Liu, M.D., M.S.

CHAPTER 1

Medical Comorbidities and Behavioral Health

Clinical Case 1

Mr. Smith is a 56-year-old man with a history of bipolar I disorder and two myocardial infarctions. His brother brought him into the emergency department with concerns of rambling speech, aggressive behavior, cough, and shortness of breath. The brother is 62 years old and does not have any past medical or psychiatric history.

1. How does Mr. Smith's severe mental illness contribute to his respiratory illness?

   A. He is 50% more likely to die from chronic obstructive pulmonary disease (COPD).
   B. He is likely to be delusional about his respiratory symptoms.
   C. He is more likely to get pneumonia and influenza.
   D. Mania tends to cause hyperventilation.

2. From the perspective of preventive medicine, why are patients with severe mental illness more likely to have respiratory problems?

   A. They are more likely to receive excessive influenza vaccines.
   B. Approximately 33% of patients with severe mental illness are tobacco smokers.
   C. They consume more than one-third of all tobacco products.
   D. They are more likely to live outside in high-humidity environments.

3. What is the most likely reason Mr. Smith has had two myocardial infarctions while his brother has not?

   A. He was at higher risk of developing metabolic syndrome and related vascular disease.
   B. He was more likely to have received an invasive cardiovascular procedure.
   C. He was more likely to have been prescribed an angiotensin-converting enzyme inhibitor.
   D. All of the above.

4. What should you consider when deciding how to treat Mr. Smith's mania?

   A. Similar weight gain is caused by either 20 mg of olanzapine or 10 mg of olanzapine.
   B. Antipsychotics vary greatly with regard to metabolic risk.
   C. Once the patient is stabilized, his medications should not be switched.
   D. Sodium valproate is a good option because it is weight neutral.
   E. All of the above.

Clinical Case 2

A 49-year-old woman with schizophrenia is found deceased in her apartment. Her medical records indicate that she was taking quetiapine and that her blood pressure readings at the mental health clinic had consistently been elevated.

1. How likely is it that the woman was prescribed antihypertensive medication?

   A. Less than 25%.
   B. Between 25% and 50%.
   C. Between 50% and 75%.
   D. More than 75%.

2. What is true about her cause of death?

   A. She is more likely to have died from suicide or injury than from natural causes.
   B. She is more likely to have died from natural causes than from suicide or injury.

C. The cause of death is unlikely to have been related to preventive medical interventions.
D. Because she had severe mental illness, she was more likely to die 5 years earlier than the general population.

3. Why could this woman have died at such a young age?

A. Her Framingham Cardiovascular Risk Score was likely similar to that of a woman 10–15 years older in the general population.
B. She was two times more likely to die as a result of diabetes.
C. She was two times more likely to die from hepatitis C.
D. None of the above.

Clinical Case 3

You were recently promoted to the position of director of a mental health clinic. You quickly discover that many of your patients have poor access to primary care.

1. Which of the following would be reasonable expectation(s) of the providers at your clinic?

A. Monitoring waist circumference of a patient after starting risperidone.
B. Following thyroid-stimulating hormone levels.
C. Checking hemoglobin A_{1c} in a patient taking a weight-neutral antipsychotic.
D. Treating those who screen positive for hepatitis C with ribavirin and interferon.
E. Answers A, B, and C.

2. Which patient may benefit most, in terms of the prevention of disability or hospitalization, from a psychiatrist's consultation with or referral to a primary care provider?

A. A high school football player who has torn his Achilles tendon and is depressed about having to stop playing sports for the season.
B. A 70-year-old woman with generalized anxiety disorder and end-stage congestive heart failure.
C. A 30-year-old woman with bipolar I disorder and hypertension.
D. A 50-year-old man with schizophrenia who has diabetes complicated by blindness and end-stage renal disease.

3. How can your clinic deliver better collaborative care?

   A. Screen for common medical conditions and refer patients to necessary services.
   B. Colocate with a financially accessible primary care office.
   C. Encourage patients to attend a free aerobics group in the local community center.
   D. All of the above.

4. Funding for which services is provided by a Medicaid-funded health home for patients with severe mental illness?

   A. Consultation with a family medicine doctor to guide the psychiatrist in screening and basic preventive care.
   B. Direct provision of comprehensive preventive care by a family medicine doctor.
   C. Case management for assessing, monitoring, coordinating, and planning for patients' physical health needs.
   D. Any of the above.
   E. Answers A and C.

CHAPTER 2

Fundamentals of Preventive Care

Clinical Case 1

Mrs. Johnson is a 55-year-old black woman with major depressive disorder, hypertension, and a 20 pack-year smoking history who sees you for a follow-up visit. She was discharged from the hospital after an acute myocardial infarction 4 weeks ago. Her discharge medications included sertraline 100 mg/day, metoprolol 25 mg bid, lisinopril 10 mg/day, atorvastatin 80 mg qhs, and aspirin 81 mg/day.

1. What is the most beneficial intervention to prevent Mrs. Johnson from having another myocardial infarction?

   A. Increase her dose of atorvastatin from 80 mg to 120 mg/day.
   B. Add lithium to adjunct selective serotonin reuptake inhibitor therapy.
   C. Counsel her on smoking cessation.
   D. Decrease the dose of sertraline to 50 mg/day.
   E. Increase the dose of aspirin to 325 mg/day.

2. What type of preventive care is provided by Mrs. Johnson's new medications?

   A. Primary prevention.
   B. Secondary prevention.
   C. Tertiary prevention.
   D. None, as she already suffered a heart attack.

3. Encouraging Mrs. Johnson to follow up with her primary care physician for routine breast cancer screening is an example of which of the following?

   A. Primary prevention.
   B. Secondary prevention.
   C. Tertiary prevention.
   D. Diagnostic testing.
   E. None of the above.

Clinical Case 2

Ms. Stevens is a 45-year-old woman who has poor follow-up with primary care. She has no personal or family history of breast cancer.

1. How often should Ms. Stevens be getting routine pap smears?

   A. She should have a pap smear every year.
   B. She should have a pap smear every 2 years.
   C. You should look for updated screening guidelines from a source such as National Guideline Clearinghouse (www.guideline.gov).
   D. This decision requires the expertise of a gynecologist.

2. You find that the USPSTF recommendation for breast cancer screening in an average 45-year-old woman is grade C. What does this mean?

   A. This service should be offered only to selected patients because the net benefit is likely to be small.
   B. This service should be discouraged because there is no net benefit or because harms outweigh the benefits.
   C. This service should be offered, and the net benefit is likely to be at least moderate.
   D. This service should be offered because the net benefit is substantial.
   E. There is insufficient evidence to offer or discourage this service.

3. You find that the USPSTF recommendation for a clinical breast examination in an average 45-year-old woman is grade I. What does this mean?

   A. This service should be offered only to selected patients because the net benefit is likely to be small.
   B. This service should be discouraged because there is no net benefit or because harms outweigh the benefits.
   C. This service should be offered, and the net benefit is likely to be at least moderate.

D. This service should be offered because the net benefit is substantial.
E. There is insufficient evidence to offer or discourage this service.

4. You find that the USPSTF recommendation for alcohol misuse screening and brief behavioral counseling is grade B. What does this mean?

    A. This service should be offered only to selected patients because the net benefit is likely to be small.
    B. This service should be discouraged because there is no net benefit or because harms outweigh the benefits.
    C. This service should be offered, and the net benefit is likely to be at least moderate.
    D. This service should be offered because the net benefit is substantial.
    E. There is insufficient evidence to offer or discourage this service.

Clinical Case 3

Mr. Carson is a 45-year-old Caucasian man with obesity, hypertension, a history of extensive smoking, and schizophrenia who is receiving olanzapine monotherapy. He comes to your office to establish psychiatric care but tells you that he has not been to a primary care doctor in years.

1. What would be a standard secondary prevention measure?

    A. Starting blood pressure medication.
    B. Adding topiramate for weight loss.
    C. Ordering a hemoglobin A_{1c} test.
    D. Administering the influenza vaccine.

2. You weigh Mr. Carson and find his body mass index to be 30 and decide to start motivational interviewing. Obesity screening is an example of which of the following?

    A. Primary prevention.
    B. Secondary prevention.
    C. Tertiary prevention.
    D. Diagnostic screening.

3. Which is essential for an effective screening program?

    A. The screening test must be able to detect the disease during a clinical stage.
    B. Screening must be able to identify a disease that becomes clinically significant if left untreated.

C. The disease in question may or may not have a cure.
D. The cost of the screening test does not matter for a potentially fatal disease.
E. If a test is 100% specific, then sensitivity does not matter when evaluating a screening program.
F. All of the above.

Clinical Case 4

You are the psychiatrist for a busy county-run clinic. Many of your patients have trouble accessing primary care doctors, and you serve as their only consistent contact with the health care system. Mr. Lee is a 30-year-old, sexually active, Asian man with a history of schizoaffective disorder and a 10 pack-year smoking history. His psychiatric symptoms have been stabilized with quetiapine and fluoxetine, and he comes to the clinic about once every 6–12 months for follow-up.

1. Which measure(s) would help prevent Mr. Lee from medical illness?

   A. Screen for HIV.
   B. Check his lipid panel.
   C. Check his hemoglobin A_{1c} level.
   D. Counsel him on smoking cessation.
   E. All of the above.

2. Which of the following measures would be considered primary prevention for Mr. Lee?

   A. Screen for HIV.
   B. Check his lipid panel.
   C. Check his hemoglobin A_{1c} level.
   D. Counsel him on smoking cessation.
   E. Answers A, B, and D.

3. How should you start preventive care screening with Mr. Lee?

   A. Implement all the preventive care interventions at one visit.
   B. Spread them over several visits.
   C. Defer them until the patient establishes with primary care.
   D. Leave it up to the patient to decide when to implement them.
   E. Answer A or B.

CHAPTER 3

Cultural Considerations in Psychiatry

Clinical Case 1

A Spanish-speaking woman has been brought to see you by a *curandero* (a traditional healer) and her bilingual husband. At a funeral that morning, she had a fit of uncontrollable screaming and shaking of her extremities that resulted in her fainting. She is asymptomatic and is currently in no distress, but her vital signs are notable for a blood pressure of 160/90. You decide to prescribe hydrochlorothiazide for the patient.

1. What consequences are more likely to occur if the patient's cultural perspective is addressed?

   A. She will experience increased stress and will be at increased risk of hypertensive emergency.
   B. She will be more likely to accept assessment and recommendations and to follow up with preventive medical care.
   C. She may be upset that her provider is not addressing her medical concerns.
   D. Answers A and B.

2. What is the best initial approach with this patient?

   A. Ask the patient what she thinks is happening.
   B. Tell her she is likely suffering from *ataque de nervios* ("attack of nerves").

C. Ask why she has not received treatment from a medical professional for her blood pressure.
D. Offer her an as-needed prescription for lorazepam.

3. What is the best approach to ensure long-term treatment of this patient's blood pressure?

A. Work together with the *curandero* to form a treatment plan.
B. Ask the patient's husband to assist with translation.
C. Discourage her from seeing a "traditional healer" for serious medical issues.
D. Warn her that she may have a stroke if she does not take medication.

Clinical Case 2

Ms. Chea, a 53-year-old Cambodian woman with a history of schizoaffective disorder, stroke, and poor medication adherence is admitted to an inpatient psychiatric facility because her aging mother is no longer able to provide the level of care Ms. Chea needs. A court order requires that she take psychiatric medication. Ms. Chea takes her oral antipsychotic and mood stabilizer, but she refuses her aspirin and statin. When you explain that she needs to take these medications to prevent a stroke, she insists that all she needs to do to be healthy is to eat traditional Cambodian food.

1. What best describes minority patients similar to Ms. Chea who have both serious mental illness and co-occurring medical issues?

A. Compared with nonminorities, they are more likely to have worse outcomes, including increased mortality.
B. They are decreasing in number because the proportion of minorities in the United States has finally stopped growing.
C. They benefit most from a multicultural approach that focuses on educating them using professional translation.
D. All of the above.

2. As the psychiatrist of Ms. Chea, how could you be more culturally conscious?

A. Reflect about how your cultural beliefs may affect treatment.
B. Educate yourself about Cambodian culture and common beliefs regarding health and illness.
C. Empathize with Ms. Chea's beliefs, even if they differ from your own.
D. All of the above.

Clinical Case 3

Mrs. Domingue is a 52-year-old Haitian immigrant with no previous mental illness who is brought to your clinic by her daughter. Since immigrating to the United States a year ago, Mrs. Domingue has become progressively more withdrawn with decreased appetite and difficulty falling asleep.

1. What might be the best initial approach to caring for Mrs. Domingue?

   A. Explore the patient's ethnic background, spiritual views, and finances.
   B. Diagnose her with major depressive disorder and prescribe sertraline 50 mg/day.
   C. Ask the patient and her daughter what could be causing her symptoms.
   D. Answers A and C.

2. Which would be the best follow-up question(s) to ask?

   A. "What have you done to cope with these problems?"
   B. "For you, what are the most important aspects of your background or identity?"
   C. "What troubles you most about your problems?"
   D. Answers A and C.
   E. Answers A, B, and C.

3. Mrs. Domingue tells you she has been possessed by a *loa* (a spirit) and wants a *houngan* (a Vodou priest) to "cure" her. How should you start treatment?

   A. Educate her on the biochemical model of depression, providing the latest evidence-based guidelines.
   B. Offer her weekly psychodynamic therapy with the help of an interpreter.
   C. Consult with a *houngan* in your community to work together to treat her depression.
   D. Provide supportive listening today so she will return when she is ready for treatment.
   E. Kindly inform her that there is no evidence that Vodou can cure disease.

CHAPTER 4

Preventive Medicine and Psychiatric Training Considerations

Clinical Case 1

You are the psychiatrist of an urban community mental health center for underserved patients. The clinic has recently accepted a contract from the county to care for a greater proportion of patients who previously did not have health insurance.

1. Which of the following is important to help your patients access preventive medical care services?

    A. Have a nurse manager on board who works closely with a primary care physician (PCP) and psychiatrist.
    B. Colocate a primary care doctor in the behavioral health clinic.
    C. Develop a referral system for medical problems.
    D. Perform basic screening and referrals to primary care.
    E. All of the above.

2. Which estimate is true about when patients with mental disorders are likely to die in relation to the general population?

    A. At about the same age.
    B. 2 years earlier.
    C. 8 years earlier.
    D. 25 years earlier.

3. Which of the following is true?

   A. Patients with depression are at higher risk for medical illness.
   B. Depression increases the risk of myocardial infarction.
   C. Earlier detection of medical illness in psychiatric patients has been shown to decrease mortality.
   D. All of the above.

Clinical Case 2

Ms. Hernandez is a 45-year-old Mexican woman with history of major depressive disorder, diabetes mellitus, obesity, and hypertension. Today her hemoglobin A_{1c} level is 10% and her Patient Health Questionnaire (PHQ-9) score is 22.

1. Which of the following models of care is best suited to help Ms. Hernandez?

   A. A PCP who refers her to a mental health clinic.
   B. A nurse manager who works with a psychiatrist and PCP in a collaborative team.
   C. A system that prevents the family physician from communicating with the psychiatrist to ensure patient privacy.
   D. Any of the above.

2. After 6 months of treatment based on the initial model, Ms. Hernandez's depression improves and her PHQ-9 score is now 5. She also has better control of her diabetes, with a hemoglobin A_{1c} level of 7%. What level of care is appropriate now?

   A. Monitoring every month by both PCP and psychiatrist.
   B. Return to primary care clinic as needed.
   C. Follow up with a nurse manager every month and a PCP every 3–6 months.
   D. Monthly visits at an endocrinology clinic.

3. Ms. Hernandez wants to transfer her care to an academic medical center. Which of the following is true about a clinic where she may receive both medical and psychiatric care from a senior psychiatry resident?

   A. This type of clinic does not yet exist.
   B. It may improve her satisfaction with care.
   C. It may improve her psychiatric symptoms but worsen her active medical problems and screening for preventive care.
   D. It would not benefit psychiatry residents.

SECTION II

Cardiovascular and Pulmonary Disorders in the Psychiatric Patient Population

Section Editor:

Glen L. Xiong, M.D.

Matthew Reed, M.D., M.S.P.H.

With

Sara Teasdale, M.D.

Christine Kho, M.D.

CHAPTER 5

Coronary Artery Disease

Clinical Case 1

Ms. Jones is a 60-year-old woman with a history of bipolar I disorder, hypertension, type 2 diabetes and dyslipidemia and a 45 pack-year smoking history who presents to the emergency room with constant substernal pressure for 1 hour. Electrocardiogram (ECG) shows ST-segment elevation, and labs reveal significantly elevated troponins. The patient is rushed to the cardiac catheterization lab, where she is found to have an occlusion of the proximal right coronary artery. A single drug-eluting stent is placed.

1. Ms. Jones's bipolar disorder is well controlled with lithium for maintenance. Which of her other medications increases her risk for lithium toxicity?

   A. Lisinopril.
   B. Metformin.
   C. Atorvastatin.
   D. Aspirin.

2. Ms. Jones should begin taking which of the following medications prior to discharge from the hospital?

   A. A short-acting dihydropyridine calcium channel blocker.
   B. Antiplatelet therapy.
   C. Supplemental vitamins B_6, B_{12}, C, and E.
   D. Hormone therapy.

3. Which of the following lifestyle modifications should be recommended to Ms. Jones for secondary prevention of CAD?

   A. Smoking cessation.
   B. Maintenance of body mass index (BMI) below 25.

C. Diet high in saturated and trans fats.
D. Routine exercise for 30–60 minutes at least 3–4 times per week.
E. Answers A and D.
F. Answers A, B, and D.

Clinical Case 2

Mr. Ames is a 70-year-old man with a history of depression, obesity, hypertension, and CAD who presents to your clinic with worsening depression. He retired from a rewarding career 4 months ago but has found it difficult to adapt to retired life. His primary care physician diagnosed him with depression and prescribed a selective serotonin reuptake inhibitor. However, before starting to take the medication, the patient sustained a myocardial infarction. Since then, he has felt even worse. He worries about his medical conditions and feels guilty that he is a burden on his wife.

1. What percentage of patients with CAD also have comorbid depressive symptoms?

   A. 5%.
   B. 20%.
   C. 40%.
   D. 75%.

2. Mr. Ames begins taking a cardioselective β-blocker after his myocardial infarction. Which of the following conditions would be considered an absolute contraindication to β-blocker use?

   A. Depression.
   B. Chronic obstructive pulmonary disease (COPD).
   C. Benign prostatic hyperplasia.
   D. Congestive heart failure (CHF).
   E. All of the above.
   F. None of the above.

3. Which of the following are potential mechanisms by which mental stress may contribute to cardiac events?

   A. Takotsubo cardiomyopathy.
   B. Sympathetic activation and vagal deactivation.
   C. Mental stress–induced myocardial ischemia.
   D. Platelet activation.
   E. All of the above.
   F. Answers B and D.

Clinical Case 3

Ms. Zimmer is a healthy 25-year-old woman with newly diagnosed schizophrenia. Her body BMI is 37, and she is concerned that she will gain more weight while taking a second-generation antipsychotic. Her mother died of a myocardial infarction at age 55, and her father has type 2 diabetes. According to the Framingham Risk Calculator, her risk for myocardial infarction in the next 10 years is less than 10%.

1. Higher rates of which modifiable risk factor(s) for CAD are seen in chronically mentally ill patients?

   A. Smoking.
   B. Diet high in saturated fats, cholesterol.
   C. Lack of exercise and sedentary lifestyle.
   D. Obesity.
   E. All of the above.

2. Which of the following variables are used as part of the Framingham risk calculator to determine 10-year risk estimates for myocardial infarction?

   A. Fasting blood sugar.
   B. Diabetes.
   C. Smoking status.
   D. Systolic blood pressure.
   E. All of the above.
   F. Answers B, C, and D.
   G. Answers C and D.

3. Which of the following parameters should be measured prior to and during treatment with second-generation antipsychotics to prevent the development of metabolic syndrome?

   A. BMI.
   B. Electrolytes.
   C. Screening ECG.
   D. Fasting plasma glucose.
   E. All of the above.
   F. Answers A and D.
   G. Answers A, C, and D.

CHAPTER 6

Hypertension

Clinical Case 1

Mr. Jameson is a 45-year-old black man with major depressive disorder and a body mass index (BMI) of 41 who presents for psychiatric follow-up. He has no contact with other medical care providers. His blood pressure is 148/92 mmHg, but his chart reveals no previous diagnosis of hypertension or history of chronic kidney disease. His blood pressure at his visit 3 months ago was 148/96 mmHg.

1. Which of the following is the most likely diagnosis for Mr. Jameson?

   A. Normal blood pressure.
   B. Prehypertension.
   C. Stage 1 hypertension.
   D. Stage 2 hypertension.
   E. Urgent hypertension.

2. Which of the following is the best treatment for Mr. Jameson's hypertension?

   A. Angiotensin-converting enzyme (ACE) inhibitor.
   B. Angiotensin receptor blocker (ARB).
   C. Calcium channel blocker (CCB).
   D. β-Blocker.
   E. Changes in diet and exercise only.

3. Which condition is most likely the cause of Mr. Jameson's hypertension?

   A. Essential or idiopathic hypertension.
   B. Medication-induced hypertension.
   C. Kidney disease.
   D. Sleep apnea.
   E. Obesity.

4. For every 20 mmHg of systolic blood pressure above 115 mmHg, there is a ______-fold increase in death from stroke and coronary artery disease (CAD).

   A. 2.
   B. 5.
   C. 6.
   D. 10.
   E. There is no increase in death from stroke and CAD.

Clinical Case 2

Mr. Neel is a 55-year-old white man with bipolar I disorder and a BMI of 38 who has returned to the clinic for psychiatric follow-up. His blood pressure was elevated at his last previous appointment 1 month ago (150/93) and is 155/92 at the current appointment. He also notes having had an elevated blood pressure when he checked it in the pharmacy 2 weeks ago. He is asymptomatic and does not have any known medical issues other than bipolar disorder and obesity. He takes lithium and had a therapeutic level (0.8 mEq/L) when the level was checked 1 month ago. His basic metabolic panel obtained at the same time was within normal limits.

1. Mr. Neel states that he is going to start exercising. How much of a reduction in his blood pressure can he expect if he engages in aerobic exercise for at least 30 minutes a day most days of the week?

   A. Up to 20 mm/Hg.
   B. 2–4 mm/Hg.
   C. 4–9 mm/Hg.
   D. None.

2. Which medication would be most appropriate to treat Mr. Neel's hypertension?

   A. Thiazide diuretic.
   B. CCB.
   C. ACE inhibitor.
   D. ARB.
   E. β-Blocker.

3. Which of the following is the correct blood pressure goal for Mr. Neel?

   A. 120/80 mmHg.
   B. Less than 150/90 mmHg.
   C. Less than 140/90 mmHg.
   D. Less than 140/80 mmHg.

CHAPTER 7

Dyslipidemia

Clinical Case 1

Mr. Helms is a 46-year-old man with hypertension and schizophrenia who presents to the clinic for psychiatric follow-up. He reports doing well with risperidone monotherapy for schizophrenia. You have encouraged him to establish care with a primary care physician to treat his blood pressure and get other age-appropriate screening. However, Mr. Helms refuses to see another physician and states that he feels fine. He is willing to continue seeing you at your clinic. You are concerned about his cardiovascular health and wonder if he has elevated cholesterol.

1. At what age does the U.S. Preventive Services Task Force (USPSTF) recommend that physicians start screening for dyslipidemia in individuals at average risk?

   A. 30 for men; 40 for women.
   B. 35 for men; 45 for women.
   C. 40 for men; 50 for women.
   D. 45 for both men and women.

2. What percentage of individuals diagnosed with both schizophrenia and dyslipidemia actually receive cholesterol-lowering treatment?

   A. <20%.
   B. 30%.
   C. 45%.
   D. 60%.
   E. >80%.

3. Which of the following laboratory studies is (are) necessary to establish a diagnosis of dyslipidemia and determine intensity of therapy?

   A. Lipid panel.
   B. Complete metabolic panel.
   C. Hemoglobin A_{1c}.
   D. Complete blood count.
   E. Answers A and C.
   F. Answers A and B.

4. On review of the electronic medical record, you notice that there are no results for previously ordered fasting lipid panels. Which of the following would be the best intervention to ensure that Mr. Helms completes his labs?

   A. Give directions to a lab near his home.
   B. Ask the family to remind the patient.
   C. Get a nonfasting lipid panel now.
   D. Refuse to schedule next appointment until labs are complete.

Clinical Case 2

Ms. Roberts is a 46-year-old nonsmoking black woman with hypertension (treated with lisinopril) and bipolar I disorder seen regularly by her psychiatrist, who notes that she has not yet been screened for dyslipidemia. He orders a nonfasting lipid panel and hemoglobin A_{1c}. He also measures her blood pressure and calculates her atherosclerotic CVD risk. The patient's results are as follows:

Total cholesterol: 257 mg/dL	Hemoglobin A_{1c}: 5.5
HDL: 47 mg/dL	Blood pressure: 150/87 mmHg
Triglycerides: 330 mg/dL	10-year atherosclerotic CVD risk: 8.5%
LDL (calculated): 145 mg/dL	

1. What is the preferred treatment for dyslipidemia if dietary and lifestyle modifications prove ineffective?

   A. Niacin.
   B. Fibrate.
   C. Bile acid sequestrants.
   D. Statin medication.

2. For this patient, which of the following measures should be used when deciding to treat and determining the intensity of treatment for dyslipidemia?

   A. Calculated LDL.
   B. Triglycerides.
   C. Hemoglobin A_{1c}.
   D. Non-HDL cholesterol.
   E. Body mass index (BMI).

3. After attempting to improve her diet and exercise regimen for more than 3 months, Ms. Roberts is unable to reduce her cholesterol by 30%. What is the next step?

   A. Begin a low- to moderate-intensity statin.
   B. Begin a moderate- to high-intensity statin.
   C. Begin a high-intensity statin.
   D. Continue lifestyle changes.

Clinical Case 3

Mr. Lewis is a nonsmoking 65-year-old white man with hypertension, grade II obesity (BMI≥35), and schizophrenia. He is seen regularly in the psychiatry clinic, and his psychiatric symptoms have been stable with olanzapine monotherapy. Today he is concerned about his risk for a stroke or heart attack. He does not have any symptoms for either condition but recently saw a commercial detailing the adverse metabolic side effects associated with olanzapine. Mr. Lewis is a nonsmoker. He has been trying to eat well and exercise more regularly but has been unable to stick with any comprehensive lifestyle and/or dietary programs over the past 6 months. His blood pressure today is 155/90, and he reports compliance taking daily hydrochlorothiazide. The results for his yearly fasting screen for dyslipidemia and diabetes, as well as his calculated 10-year atherosclerotic CVD risk, are as follows:

Total cholesterol: 290 mg/dL	Hemoglobin A_{1c}: 5.4
HDL: 45 mg/dL	Blood pressure: 155/90 mmHg
Triglycerides: 250 mg/dL	10-year atherosclerotic CVD risk: 27.0%
LDL (calculated): 196 mg/dL	

1. Which further assessment should take place before a treatment option for Mr. Lewis's dyslipidemia is chosen?

   A. Waist circumference.
   B. Skinfold thickness.
   C. Secondary causes of hyperlipidemia.
   D. Fasting glucose.

2. Which of the following treatment interventions is now indicated?

   A. An antipsychotic that has lower risk of metabolic syndrome.
   B. A moderate-intensity statin.
   C. A high-intensity statin.
   D. Water aerobics.

3. Should changing Mr. Lewis's antipsychotic not result in a 30%–50% reduction in cholesterol, which of the following statin medications should be tried?

   A. Pravastatin.
   B. Atorvastatin.
   C. Rosuvastatin.
   D. Answer B or C.
   E. Answer A, B, or C.

CHAPTER 8

Tobacco Dependence

Clinical Case 1

Mrs. Mackey is a 57-year-old woman with schizoaffective disorder, chronic obstructive pulmonary disease, obesity, and tobacco dependence since age 18 who returns to the clinic for routine psychiatric follow-up. She reports good compliance with olanzapine, which has been effective in controlling auditory hallucinations and episodes of mania. It has been over a year since her last psychiatric hospitalization. She also denies current depressive symptoms and suicidal ideation. Mrs. Mackey is more frequently short of breath with exertion, and she attributes this to smoking. She expresses interest in smoking cessation.

1. Why would Mrs. Mackey, an individuals with a serious mental illness, have an increased risk for nicotine dependence?

   A. Abnormalities in nicotinic receptors.
   B. Antidepressant properties of nicotine.
   C. Exposure to tobacco in treatment environments.
   D. All of the above.
   E. Answers A and C only.

2. Smoking rates in the general population have declined by 50% over the past 50 years. How much have the rates declined among the seriously mentally ill?

   A. 40%.
   B. 25%.

C. 15%.
D. Rates have not declined.

3. What is the most effective treatment option available for Mrs. Mackey's nicotine dependence?

   A. Smoking cessation medications.
   B. Psychosocial treatments.
   C. Combined treatment with medications and psychosocial treatments.
   D. Psychodynamic psychotherapy.

4. Which smoking cessation medication would likely provide the most benefit for Mrs. Mackey?

   A. Nicotine replacement.
   B. Bupropion.
   C. Nortriptyline.
   D. Varenicline.

Clinical Case 2

Mrs. Peters is an overweight 45-year-old woman with major depressive disorder and tobacco dependence who presents for a medication management appointment and asks about smoking cessation. She reports that since she started taking paroxetine for major depressive disorder, she has gained 10 lbs, and she worries that she will gain more weight if she stops smoking.

1. The following exchange demonstrates which psychotherapeutic technique?

   Mental health provider: I see. Smoking has been a real benefit for your weight management.
   Patient: Yes, but it has also caused me a lot of problems.
   Mental health provider: Really? Like what?
   Patient: I mean…my clothes always stink, my husband wants me to stop, and I am worried I am going to get cancer.

   A. Psychoeducation.
   B. Problem solving.
   C. Cognitive-behavioral therapy.
   D. Motivational interviewing.

2. Approximately how much weight could Mrs. Peters expect to gain after she stops smoking?

   A. 2 lbs.
   B. 5 lbs.
   C. 10 lbs.
   D. 20 lbs.

3. Which smoking cessation medication would likely be of most benefit for Mrs. Peters?

   A. Nicotine replacement.
   B. Bupropion.
   C. Nortriptyline.
   D. Varenicline.

CHAPTER 9

Chronic Obstructive Pulmonary Disease

Clinical Case 1

Mr. Kelso is a 54-year-old man with schizoaffective disorder who presents to your county clinic to establish care after moving in with his sister a few months ago. He has been stable on clozapine for many years. He denies any ongoing medical issues but has a mild cough throughout the encounter. His sister notes that he is quite sedentary and wheezes whenever he exerts himself. He has a 60 pack-year smoking history but has cut down dramatically since moving in with her. He smokes half a pack per day and with his sister's help plans to stop completely.

1. You suspect that Mr. Kelso might have chronic obstructive pulmonary disease (COPD). How would you confirm the diagnosis?

   A. History.
   B. Physical examination.
   C. Spirometry.
   D. Imaging studies.

2. Mr. Kelso is sent for pulmonary function studies. His ratio of forced expiratory volume after 1 second (FEV_1) to forced vital capacity (FVC) is 0.6, and his FEV_1 is 72%. What do you conclude from these results?

   A. He has COPD.
   B. He does not have COPD.
   C. Findings are indeterminate.
   D. Additional imaging is needed.

3. What is the most important therapeutic intervention for COPD?

   A. Short-acting bronchodilators.
   B. Long-acting bronchodilators.
   C. Smoking cessation.
   D. Inhaled corticosteroids.

4. What are potential adverse effects of smoking cessation?

   A. Psychiatric decompensation.
   B. Weight gain.
   C. Clozapine toxicity.
   D. Answers B and C.
   E. Answers A, B, and C.

Clinical Case 2

Ms. Lane is a 64-year-old woman with COPD, obesity, and schizophrenia who was brought into the clinic by her group home operator who is concerned that the patient is not sleeping at night and is bothering her roommates. Ms. Lane requests a prescription for lorazepam as needed to help her sleep. On evaluation, Ms. Lane complains of a cough, and she believes that her roommates are somehow making her cough worse because they do not like her. Ms. Lane's chronic cough has worsened over the past few months, and she has become more short of breath with activity. She takes salmeterol, a long-acting inhaled β_2-agonist, plus as-needed albuterol/ipratropium for COPD.

1. Which of the following would be the most appropriate management choice for Ms. Lane's insomnia?

   A. Lorazepam.
   B. Increased perphenazine.
   C. Acetaminophen with codeine.
   D. Referral to a primary care provider.

2. Ms. Lane's primary care provider prescribed an inhaled corticosteroid to complement the patient's long-acting β_2-agonist and short-acting bronchodilator. However, at her next appointment with you, Ms. Lane's cough has not improved. What is the best next step in management?

   A. Start theophylline.
   B. Start a long-acting anticholinergic.
   C. Call the group home operator to verify compliance.

D. Refer to a pulmonologist.
E. All of the above.

3. Which of the following immunization(s) should be offered to Ms. Lane?

A. Measles, mumps, rubella (MMR).
B. Tetanus.
C. Pneumonia.
D. Influenza.
E. Answers C and D.

SECTION III

Endocrine and Metabolic Disorders in the Psychiatric Patient Population

Section Editor:

Craig R. Keenan, M.D.

Lindsey Enoch, M.D.

With

Julie Hylton, M.D.

Stephany Sanchez, M.D.

CHAPTER 10

Diabetes

Clinical Case 1

Ms. Amber is a 45-year-old woman who comes into your office to establish care for depression. She describes low mood, anhedonia, fatigue, increased appetite and thirst, and weight gain. She is not taking any medication at this time, but imipramine had been helpful for her depression in the past. Her family history is remarkable for a mother and sister with diabetes. Her blood pressure is 130/70 mmHg, pulse 80 bpm, weight 150 lbs, and body mass index (BMI) 29.3.

1. What is the most appropriate next step for Ms. Amber?

    A. Start low-dose imipramine, because it has been effective in the past.
    B. Start a selective serotonin reuptake inhibitor (SSRI) and follow-up in 1 month.
    C. Start an SSRI and check hemoglobin A_{1c} (HbA_{1c}).
    D. Start an SSRI and an antihypertensive medication.

You prescribe fluoxetine 20 mg/day. When Ms. Amber returns for her 1-month follow-up, her blood pressure is 133/75 mmHg, pulse 82 bpm, and weight 152 lbs. Her HbA_{1c} value is 6.4%.

2. Which is the correct diagnosis?

    A. Type 2 diabetes.
    B. Type 1 diabetes.
    C. Normal glucose tolerance.
    D. Prediabetes.

Clinical Case 2

Mr. Beal is a 41-year-old black man with type 2 diabetes, osteoarthritis, and schizoaffective disorder. He is currently taking metformin 500 mg bid, risperidone 2 mg bid, and lithium 450 mg bid. He admits to occasionally missing doses of his medications. He reports some blurry vision but otherwise has no acute complaints. His blood pressure today is 167/95 mmHg, pulse 72 bpm, and BMI 31.2. Two months ago, his HbA_{1c} was 7.9%, glucose level was 200 mg/dL, and basal metabolic panel was unremarkable.

1. Which of the following would be an appropriate treatment plan for this patient?

   A. Increase metformin to 1,000 mg bid and continue checking HbA_{1c} annually.
   B. Increase metformin to 2,000 mg bid and continue checking HbA_{1c} annually.
   C. Increase metformin to 1,000 mg bid and check HbA_{1c} every 3 months.
   D. Continue current dose of metformin and continue to check HbA_{1c} annually as long as it remains less than 8%.

2. In addition to checking HbA_{1c}, which of the following screening tests would you recommend for this patient with type 2 diabetes?

   A. Dilated comprehensive eye examinations every year.
   B. Urine albumin and creatinine and basic metabolic panel every year.
   C. Foot exam every year.
   D. Lipid panel every year.
   E. All of the above.

3. Mr. Beal returns to the clinic a month later. His blood pressure is 155/92 mmHg, pulse 84, and BMI 31.2. Which of the following is the most appropriate next step in management of this patient's blood pressure?

   A. Continue to monitor because his blood pressure is going down without intervention.
   B. Start metoprolol 12.5 mg bid to target a blood pressure of <140/90 mmHg.
   C. Start lisinopril 10 mg/day to target a blood pressure of <140/90 mmHg.
   D. Start hydrochlorothiazide 25 mg/day to target a blood pressure of <130/80 mmHg.

Clinical Case 3

Ms. Cathol, a 40-year-old woman with bipolar II disorder and hyperlipidemia, comes to the clinic for assessment of her bipolar medication management. She is homeless, often misses appointments, and does not have a primary care doctor. She is currently taking valproic acid 1,000 mg bid and olanzapine 10 mg hs. She feels that her medications are effective and she has not been hospitalized since starting this regimen, but she is concerned about medication side effects. She admits to minimal physical activity and eating mostly fast food. She is also drinking more soda because she is constantly thirsty and urinating often. Her blood pressure is 116/80 mmHg, pulse 76 bpm, weight 207 lbs, and BMI 34.3. Her weight was 190 lbs prior to starting olanzapine 1 year ago.

1. Which of the following is true?

   A. All second-generation antipsychotics (SGAs) result in weight gain.
   B. Olanzapine can increase risk for diabetes.
   C. This patient does not have symptoms of glucose intolerance.
   D. Weight loss is unlikely to prevent this patient from developing diabetes.

2. Which of the following would be the most appropriate therapy for this patient?

   A. Stop the olanzapine and start ziprasidone.
   B. Recommend weight loss.
   C. Start metformin 500 mg/day.
   D. All of the above.

CHAPTER 11

Obesity

Clinical Case 1

Mr. Damons is a 42-year-old man with schizophrenia, posttraumatic stress disorder, hyperlipidemia, and hypertension who presents to the clinic to establish care. He recently moved from out of state and has not been able to see a doctor or get medications for 3 months. He is unsure of his most recent medications but has taken olanzapine, aripiprazole, and lithium in the past. His family history is notable for depression and diabetes in both parents. Today his blood pressure is 134/83 mmHg, pulse 90 bpm, weight 275 lbs, and body mass index (BMI) 36.3. He is interested in resuming medications for his schizophrenia.

1. Which of the following is true?

   A. Approximately half of the adult population is obese.
   B. The prevalence of obesity in patients with serious mental illness is equal to that in the general population.
   C. As a class, antipsychotics are associated with more weight gain than mood stabilizers or antidepressants.
   D. Obesity is diagnosed when BMI is greater than 35.

You inform the patient of your concern about his weight gain and that based on his BMI, he is obese. You start him on aripiprazole. He returns to the clinic after 1 month.

2. Which of the following tests or vital signs are most appropriate to monitor in this patient?

   A. Thigh and waist circumferences at every visit.
   B. Lipid panels every 3 months.
   C. Waist circumference and BMI at every visit.
   D. Waist circumference annually and BMI at regular intervals.

3. Which of the following is an appropriate strategy for weight loss in this patient?

   A. Recommend reducing caloric intake by 500–1,000 calories per day.
   B. Recommend bariatric surgery.
   C. Recommend strict adherence to a low-fat diet.
   D. Recommend walking 30 minutes, 5 days a week, at a pace of 4 mph.

Clinical Case 2

Mr. Tatum is a 31-year-old man with depression and nicotine dependence, presenting for his 3-month follow-up. He complains of a 14-lb weight gain since he began taking mirtazapine at his last visit. He has been obese most of his life. He has multiple family members with diabetes and coronary artery disease. He reports good mood but feels fatigued, lethargic, and unmotivated to lose weight. Today his blood pressure is 110/76 mmHg, pulse 89 bpm, weight 260 lbs, and BMI 35.

1. Which of the following would be the most appropriate next step in addressing Mr. Tatum's obesity?

   A. Check thyroid-stimulating hormone (TSH), liver function tests (LFTs), lipid panel, and hemoglobin A_{1c}.
   B. Switch mirtazapine to paroxetine.
   C. Explore his diet and exercise habits.
   D. Both A and C.
   E. All of the above.

Mr. Tatum has his blood work done and then returns to see you after 2 weeks. His blood pressure on this day is 123/81 mmHg, his pulse is 79 bpm, and his weight and BMI are unchanged. His hemoglobin A_{1c} is 7.9%; his TSH, LFTs, and lipid panel are within normal limits.

2. Based on this information, which of the following medications would you prescribe?

   A. Metformin.
   B. Topiramate.
   C. Lisinopril.
   D. Insulin.

3. Which of the following is *not* a common side effect of metformin?

   A. Hypoglycemia.
   B. Nausea.
   C. Diarrhea.
   D. Metallic taste.

4. Which of the following medications/medication classes is also associated with weight gain?

   A. Penicillin.
   B. α-Agonists.
   C. β-Agonists.
   D. Antihistamines.

CHAPTER 12

Metabolic Syndrome

Clinical Case 1

Mrs. Seits is a 52-year-old woman with schizophrenia, hypertension, seasonal allergies, and type 2 diabetes who is presenting for routine follow-up. Her schizophrenia is well controlled with risperidone 3 mg bid. She also takes lisinopril 10 mg/day, aspirin 81 mg/day, and metformin 500 mg bid. Today her blood pressure is 130/78 mmHg, pulse 65 bpm, weight 180 lbs, and body mass index (BMI) 33. She would like to discuss the blood work you recently ordered, which had these results: hemoglobin A_{1c} 7.2%, low-density lipoprotein (LDL) 200 mg/dL, triglycerides (TG) 190 mg/dL, high-density lipoprotein (HDL) 40 mg/dL, and fasting glucose 110mg/dL. Her thyroid-stimulating hormone (TSH), liver tests, and creatinine are all within normal limits.

1. Which of the following is *not* a criterion for metabolic syndrome?

   A. Abdominal obesity.
   B. Hypertriglyceridemia.
   C. Elevated LDL.
   D. Elevated blood pressure.
   E. Impaired fasting glucose.

2. What would be the most appropriate addition to this patient's medication regimen, given the above information?

   A. Low-dose insulin at night.
   B. Simvastatin 40 mg/day.
   C. Losartan 25 mg/day.
   D. Topiramate 200 mg bid.

3. Which of the following lists specifies the correct monitoring for a patient with metabolic syndrome 12 weeks after starting a second-generation antipsychotic?

   A. BMI, blood pressure, lipid panel, and fasting glucose.
   B. Waist circumference, blood pressure, and lipid panel.
   C. BMI, blood pressure, TSH, and lipid panel.
   D. BMI, blood pressure, and lipid panel.

4. Which of the following statements about ACE inhibitors is false?

   A. They are appropriate first-line treatment for patients with high blood pressure and diabetes.
   B. They are unlikely to affect lithium levels.
   C. They can cause severe hyperkalemia.
   D. Cough is the most common side effect.

Clinical Case 2

Mrs. Heater is a 40-year-old woman who has been seeing you for schizophrenia for the last year. You have been titrating her dose of paliperidone, and she has been stable for the last 3 months. She has no known past medical history, but you notice that she has gained 40 lbs since starting paliperidone. Today her blood pressure is 160/84 mmHg, pulse 75 bpm, weight 250 lbs, BMI 34, and waist circumference 38 inches. Her lab results are as follows: fasting blood glucose 114 mg/dL, LDL 175 mg/dL, HDL 32 mg/dL, and triglycerides 210 mg/dL. Her basic metabolic panel, liver tests, and TSH are all normal.

1. Which of the following intervention(s) would be appropriate for addressing this patient's metabolic syndrome?

   A. Switching to a first-generation antipsychotic.
   B. Referral to a primary care physician (PCP).
   C. Referral to a nutritionist.
   D. All of the above.

2. Because the patient describes adverse reactions to various first-generation antipsychotics, you decide to switch the paliperidone to aripiprazole. Which of the following treatments would *not* be appropriate for this patient?

   A. Starting lisinopril 10 mg once daily.
   B. Starting metformin 500 mg bid.

C. Starting a regular walking regimen.
D. Starting simvastatin 80 mg hs.

3. Mrs. Heater returns to the clinic after 1 month. She is now taking lisinopril 10 mg/day, simvastatin 40 mg/day, metformin 500 mg bid, and aripiprazole 10 mg/day. She is no longer taking paliperidone. She thinks you are doing a great job and does not want to go to a PCP. Today her blood pressure is 184/107 mmHg, pulse 80 bpm, weight 246 lbs, and BMI 34. Her fasting blood glucose is 201 mg/dL. You ask her to return to the clinic in 1 day so you can recheck her blood pressure. On the following day her blood pressure is 190/102 mmHg. What is the most appropriate next step?

   A. Increase her to lisinopril 20 mg and have her follow up in 1 month.
   B. Discuss the importance of primary care and place another referral for a PCP.
   C. Check her waist circumference.
   D. Check another lipid panel.

4. Mrs. Heater returns for a 3-month follow-up. She says she is feeling much better now that her new PCP has adjusted her blood pressure and diabetes medications. She reports heavy snoring and daytime sleepiness at times. She is now taking lisinopril 40 mg/day, hydrochlorothiazide 25 mg/day, metformin 1,000 mg bid, glipizide 5 mg/day, simvastatin 40 mg/day, and aripiprazole 10 mg/day. Today her blood pressure is 138/71 mmHg, pulse 78 bpm, weight 230 lbs, and BMI 33. Her lab work from the day prior had these results: hemoglobin A_{1c} 6.4%, LDL 90 mg/dL, HDL 50 mg/dL, triglycerides 133 mg/dL, and normal BMP. What is the most appropriate next step?

   A. Continue current therapy.
   B. Refer for a sleep study.
   C. Change simvastatin to atorvastatin for better lipid control.
   D. Add amlodipine for blood pressure control.

CHAPTER 13

Osteoporosis

Clinical Case 1

Ms. Chen is a 51-year-old postmenopausal Asian woman who has a history of schizophrenia and is taking antipsychotic medications. She presents for psychiatric follow-up. She is doing well and has no acute complaints. Her blood pressure is 124/74 mmHg, and she weighs 120 lbs. Her updated family history shows that her mother had a hip fracture at age 65. Ms. Chen currently smokes half a pack of cigarettes per day and has a 20 pack-year smoking history. She does not drink alcohol. She had a dual-energy X-ray absorptiometry (DEXA) to determine her bone mineral density; her T-score is −1.9.

1. Which of the following is the most likely diagnosis for Ms. Chen?

   A. Normal bone density.
   B. Osteopenia.
   C. Osteoporosis.
   D. Severe osteoporosis.

2. A DEXA measures bone mineral density and yields a T-score, which is determined by which of the following?

   A. A comparison to bone mineral density of an age-, ethnicity-, and sex-matched reference.
   B. A comparison to bone mineral density of a healthy 30-year-old female reference.
   C. A comparison to bone mineral density of a healthy 30-year-old male reference.
   D. A comparison to bone mineral density of an age-matched reference.

3. Which of the following risk factor(s) does Ms. Chen have for the development of osteoporosis?

   A. Diagnosis of schizophrenia.
   B. Use of antipsychotic medication.
   C. Weight less than 126 lbs.
   D. Tobacco use.
   E. Asian race.
   F. Family history of hip fracture.
   G. All of the above.

4. Antipsychotic medications may impact bone metabolism by causing which of the following?

   A. Hypercalcemia.
   B. Hypoprolactinemia.
   C. Hyperprolactinemia.
   D. Increased vitamin D metabolism.
   E. Decreased vitamin D metabolism.

Clinical Case 2

Ms. Raynaud is a 59-year-old woman with history of depression who presents to your office for follow-up. She is taking sertraline, and her clinical depression has been controlled for the past 6 months. She mentions new-onset midline lower back pain. Ms. Raynaud denies any trauma or falls preceding the onset of her lower back pain. Physical examination reveals pinpoint tenderness along the lumbar spine. Plain films reveal a wedge deformity consistent with fracture in lumbar vertebra L2. There is no clear explanation for development of this fracture. Vitamin D level was obtained, and results show 35 ng/mL. A DEXA was ordered and revealed a T-score of −1.3.

1. What is the most likely diagnosis for Ms. Raynaud?

   A. Osteoporosis.
   B. Osteopenia.
   C. Normal bone density.
   D. Vitamin D deficiency.

2. The best pharmacological treatment for this condition would be:

   A. Calcium supplementation alone.
   B. Vitamin D supplementation alone.

C. Calcium and vitamin D supplementation.
D. Bisphosphonate alone.
E. Bisphosphonate and supplementation with calcium and vitamin D.

3. The most appropriate dosages of calcium and vitamin D supplementation for Ms. Raynaud are:

   A. Calcium 1,000 mg/day and vitamin D 400–600 IU/day.
   B. Calcium 1,200 mg/day but no additional vitamin D.
   C. Calcium 1,200 mg/day and vitamin D 800 IU/day.
   D. Calcium 1,200 mg/day and vitamin D 50,000 IU/week.

CHAPTER 14

Thyroid Disorders

Clinical Case 1

Ms. Lapperstein is a 34-year-old woman with a known history of depression and hypertension. Her depression had been well controlled for over a year with sertraline 100 mg/day. She presents to your office today reporting low moods and fatigue for the past 6 weeks. She has gained 12 lbs during that time. She also notes often feeling cold. Today, her blood pressure is 130/76 mmHg, pulse 54 bpm, weight 174 lbs, and body mass index (BMI) 33. Review of family history reveals that Ms. Lapperstein's mother had an unspecified thyroid disease. You check her thyroid-stimulating hormone (TSH) level, which returns elevated.

1. In addition to the above-named symptoms, which of the following is a common symptom of hypothyroidism?

   A. Tremor.
   B. Frequent bowel movements.
   C. Constipation.
   D. Heart palpitations.

2. Free thyroxine (free T_4) testing returned at a low value, confirming the diagnosis of hypothyroidism. No palpable masses were found on physical examination. What is an appropriate initial treatment plan for Ms. Lapperstein?

   A. Start levothyroxine 12 μg/day and measure serum TSH 2 weeks after initiating treatment.
   B. Start levothyroxine 25 μg/day and measure serum TSH 6–8 weeks after initiating treatment.

C. Order a follow-up serum TSH in 4 weeks but do not initiate a medication at this time.
D. Start levothyroxine 150 μg/day and measure serum TSH 12 weeks after initiating treatment.

Clinical Case 2

Ms. Gamble is a 66-year-old woman with history of hyperlipidemia and gastroesophageal reflux disease (GERD) who was referred to you at the suggestion of her daughter for a chief complaint of lethargy over the past 2 months, which her family suspects is related to depression. The patient has no psychiatric history and denies ever experiencing fatigue of this nature before. She denies significant anhedonia or frequent low moods. Upon further review of systems, she endorses subjective report of racing heart, as well as mild weight loss over the last 3 months, despite normal appetite. Today her blood pressure is 137/91 mmHg, pulse 91 bpm, weight 112 lbs, and BMI 19.9.

1. Which of the following is a current guideline related to thyroid disorders?

   A. Measure serum TSH in any patient over age 35 and every 5 years thereafter, particularly in women and elderly patients.
   B. For elderly patients with any new or worsening mood symptoms or cognitive dysfunction, measure serum TSH to assess for thyroid disease.
   C. For all psychiatric patients, measure a baseline serum TSH level as part of initial workup.
   D. All of the above.

2. One-third of elderly patients with thyroid disease present with only the constellation of symptoms known as "apathetic hyperthyroidism," which includes apathy, tachycardia, and which of the following?

   A. Diarrhea.
   B. Tremor.
   C. Weight loss.
   D. Muscle weakness.

Clinical Case 3

Mr. Faber is a 29-year-old man with no significant medical history who presents to your office to establish care after a recent move to the area. He reports symptoms of depression for the past 3 months following a divorce. He also endorses symptoms consistent with a manic episode 2 years ago. You diagnose bipolar disorder and recommend starting a mood stabilizer.

1. Which of the following psychiatric medications is known to impact thyroid hormone levels?

   A. Lithium.
   B. Lamotrigine.
   C. Valproic acid.
   D. All of the above.

2. If Mr. Faber had reported a history of autoimmune thyroid disease such as Hashimoto's thyroiditis, all of the following would be necessary labs to obtain prior to lithium initiation *except:*

   A. Free T_4.
   B. Antithyroid peroxidase antibody.
   C. Erythrocyte sedimentation rate (ESR).
   D. TSH.

3. Mr. Faber begins taking lithium, which is titrated slowly over the next several months. His bipolar depression stabilizes, and he reports much improved social and work functioning. He continues to do well over the next year. At that time, however, Mr. Faber presents for a regular follow-up reporting increasing lethargy, cold intolerance, and constipation. Repeat TSH confirms hypothyroidism. What is the most appropriate course of action?

   A. Discontinue lithium and initiate an alternative mood stabilizer.
   B. Continue lithium and initiate levothyroxine 25 μg/day.
   C. Continue lithium and repeat a TSH in 2 months to determine whether further workup is necessary.
   D. Discontinue lithium and do not start an alternative agent given remission of his bipolar disorder.

SECTION IV

Infectious Disorders in the Psychiatric Patient Population

Section Editor:
Craig R. Keenan, M.D.

Chinonyerem J. Okwara, M.D.
With
George K. Gallardo, M.D.
Heather A. Vierra, M.D.

CHAPTER 15

Adult Immunizations

Clinical Case 1

Mr. Pope, a 66-year-old man with a history of bipolar II disorder, chronic kidney disease stage IV, type 2 diabetes mellitus, and hypertension, presents to your office to establish care after moving to the area. His bipolar disorder is well controlled on lithium monotherapy. The patient does not have a primary care doctor and says he will not be getting one in the next 6 months due to insurance reasons. The patient had his last tetanus booster at age 50.

1. Which of the following is the most appropriate course of action for Mr. Pope's pneumococcal vaccine?

   A. Do nothing, because pneumococcal vaccine is not indicated for this patient.
   B. Administer pneumococcal polysaccharide (PPSV23) today; revaccination is unnecessary.
   C. Administer PPSV23 today and revaccinate in 5 years.
   D. Administer pneumococcal conjugate 13-valent vaccine (PCV13) today and revaccinate in 5 years.
   E. Administer PCV13 today and have him return in 8 weeks for PPSV23.

2. Which of the following is true regarding pneumococcal vaccination?

   A. Pneumococcal vaccination reduces the rate of pneumonia in a population.
   B. Pneumococcal vaccine does not reduce the rate of pneumonia but does reduce the burden of bacteremia associated with pneumonia.

C. Only adults over age 65 should be vaccinated against pneumococcus.
D. Pneumococcal vaccination is contraindicated in patients with HIV.

3. Which of the following is correct regarding vaccinating Mr. Pope against tetanus?

A. He should receive a tetanus and diphtheria (Td) booster today and again in 10 years.
B. He should receive a tetanus, diphtheria, and pertussis vaccine (Tdap) today and return for a Td booster in 4 weeks.
C. He should receive Tdap today and have a Td booster in 10 years.
D. He does not require tetanus vaccine.

Clinical Case 2

Mr. Spaulding is a 60-year-old man with chronic depression and type 2 diabetes mellitus who presents for follow-up of his depression. The patient has not seen a primary care physician in 20 years but was diagnosed with type 2 diabetes mellitus 6 months ago while hospitalized for suicidal ideation. You have been managing his diabetes, which is easily controlled with metformin. Mr. Spaulding says he has never received hepatitis vaccinations. His physical examination is unremarkable. He denies intravenous drug use history and is sexually active only with women. He has no significant travel history and is unemployed.

1. Which of the following is correct regarding the appropriate hepatitis vaccinations for Mr. Spaulding?

A. He requires vaccinations against hepatitis A and hepatitis B.
B. He does not require any vaccination against hepatitis A or B.
C. He should be vaccinated against hepatitis B only.
D. He should be vaccinated against hepatitis A only.

2. Which of the following is correct regarding varicella zoster vaccination for Mr. Spaulding?

A. He should be tested for immunity to varicella zoster prior to receiving the vaccine.
B. He should receive the varicella zoster vaccine today.
C. He does not require vaccination against varicella zoster.
D. Varicella zoster vaccine is contraindicated in this patient.

3. Which of the following patients should *not* receive the varicella zoster vaccine?

   A. A 65-year-old man with AIDS.
   B. A 60-year-old woman with lupus on chronic prednisone therapy.
   C. A 52-year-old man on chemotherapy for lymphoma.
   D. All of the above.

Clinical Case 3

Mr. Perry is a 22-year-old man with uncontrolled bipolar I disorder with frequent manic episodes who presents to your office for an initial consultation. His last manic episode was about 1 month ago, during which time he had multiple sexual encounters with both women and men. He occasionally uses condoms. The only vaccine he recalls receiving is a Tdap at age 18.

1. Which of the following is correct regarding vaccination for Mr. Perry?

   A. He should be vaccinated against human papilloma virus (HPV).
   B. He should receive a Tdap today.
   C. He should receive pneumococcal vaccination once today and have a repeat vaccination in 5 years.
   D. Aside from an annual influenza vaccination, he does not require any vaccinations.

2. Mr. Perry should also be vaccinated against which of the following?

   A. Varicella zoster.
   B. Pneumococcus.
   C. Hepatitis B.
   D. Tdap.

3. Upon further evaluation, you find that Mr. Perry is HIV positive. Which of the following vaccines are contraindicated?

   A. Pneumococcal.
   B. Hepatitis A.
   C. Varicella zoster.
   D. HPV.

CHAPTER 16

Sexually Transmitted Infections

Clinical Case 1

Ms. Herring is a 30-year-old woman with schizoaffective disorder who presents to your office for follow-up. During the sexual history, she discloses that she occasionally engages in sex for money. She denies any dysuria or vaginal discharge. You are concerned about her overall health and realize that she is at high risk for acquiring a sexually transmitted infection (STI).

1. Ms. Herring should be screened yearly for all of the following STIs *except:*

   A. HIV.
   B. Trichomoniasis.
   C. Syphilis.
   D. Gonorrhea.

2. You discover that Ms. Herring is positive for gonorrhea. Which of the following is the best treatment for her?

   A. Single 1-g dose of oral azithromycin.
   B. Single 250-mg dose of intramuscular ceftriaxone.
   C. Single 2-g dose of oral metronidazole.
   D. Single 1-g dose of oral azithromycin and single 250-mg dose of intramuscular ceftriaxone.

3. Which of the following statements is correct?

   A. The patient should be urgently referred to a specialist for further treatment.
   B. The patient should abstain from sexual activity for 1 month after treatment.
   C. This case must be reported to public health authorities, and the patient should abstain from sex for at least 1 week.
   D. This patient's partners do not need to be treated.

Clinical Case 2

Mr. Hill is a 40-year-old man with severe depression who presents to your office for a "male problem." The patient is obviously uncomfortable when you walk into the room. Avoiding eye contact, he says that he had unprotected sex with a woman 3 weeks ago and now has developed a painless lesion on his penis. Vital signs are within normal limits. Physical examination reveals a 1-cm ulcer on his penis.

1. What is the most likely diagnosis for Mr. Hill?

   A. Gonorrhea.
   B. Herpes simplex virus.
   C. Primary syphilis.
   D. Chlamydia.

2. What is the most appropriate next step in Mr. Hill's treatment?

   A. Request rapid plasma regain (RPR) test or Venereal Disease Research Laboratory (VDRL) test for diagnosis.
   B. Treat with acyclovir 400 mg tid for 7 days.
   C. Treat with benzathine penicillin 1.44 g intramuscularly once.
   D. No treatment is required at this stage.

3. You tell Mr. Hill about your treatment plan, but he reports that as a child he had a severe reaction to penicillin he received for strep throat and required hospitalization. Which of the following is the best course of action?

   A. Continue with penicillin therapy, which is unlikely to cause the same reaction he previously had as a child.
   B. Refer this patient to an infectious disease specialist.
   C. Prescribe a reduced dose of penicillin to prevent allergic reaction.
   D. Do not treat his syphilis, because the risk is too high for this patient.

Clinical Case 3

Mr. Rush is a 20-year-old male college student who presents to the student health clinic for test-related anxiety. He complains of palpitations, insomnia, and excessive worry prior to examinations. He denies any drug use. He lives in a dorm room, and his anxiety is making it difficult for him to sustain relationships. He is sexually active with women and usually uses condoms. The only vaccination he received as a teenager was Tdap. He has no complaints aside from anxiety. Physical examination reveals multiple painful ulcers on his penis that began 2 days ago, and he states that they have appeared previously. His vital signs are normal.

1. Which of the following statements is correct?

   A. He should receive the pneumococcal vaccine.
   B. He should receive the meningococcal vaccine.
   C. He should receive the hepatitis A vaccine.
   D. He should receive a tetanus booster.

2. What would be the best treatment option for Mr. Rush's vesicular lesions?

   A. A one-time dose of azithromycin 1 g orally and ceftriaxone 250 mg intramuscularly.
   B. Doxycycline 100 mg bid for 10 days.
   C. Acyclovir 400 mg tid for 7 days.
   D. Benzathine penicillin 1.44 g intramuscularly once.

CHAPTER 17

Viral Hepatitis

Clinical Case 1

Mr. Cunningham is a 66-year-old man with a history of coronary artery disease, who underwent a three-vessel coronary artery bypass graft surgery 4 months ago. Since his surgery, he has presented to the emergency department four times for chest pain but was not diagnosed with acute coronary syndrome. His cardiologist and emergency room physician are concerned that the patient may have an anxiety disorder and referred him to you for psychiatric consultation. Mr. Cunningham has never seen a psychiatrist and does not have a primary care physician.

1. According to the revised U.S. Preventive Services Task Force (USPSTF) guidelines published in June 2013, which of the following best describes screening recommendations for hepatitis C (HCV) infection?

   A. Screen all adults older than age 18 years regardless of risk factors.
   B. Screen asymptomatic or low-risk adults one time if they were born after 1992.
   C. Screen asymptomatic or low-risk adults one time if they were born between 1945 and 1965.
   D. Screen only adults with complaints of right upper quadrant pain.

2. Mr. Cunningham tells you that he used intravenous heroin for several years but has been in full remission for 10 years. You discern that based on his age and risk factors, he should be screened for both hepatitis B (HBV) and HCV. Which of the following is the most appropriate initial screening lab for HCV?

   A. HCV RNA load.
   B. HCV genotype.

C. Anti-HCV antibody.
D. Serum transaminases.

3. Mr. Cunningham's serology tests are back, and you note that his test results are consistent with chronic HCV infection and that his HBV serology test results are all negative, including anti-HBV surface antibody. You would like to offer him appropriate vaccinations. Which of the following viruses have available vaccinations that should be offered to this patient?

   A. Hepatitis B (HBV).
   B. Hepatitis C (HCV).
   C. Hepatitis D (HDV).
   D. Hepatitis E (HEV).

4. You have been seeing Mr. Cunningham for 6 months. He is up to date on his vaccinations. He informs you today that he finally has an appointment to see the hepatologist for his chronic HCV. You anticipate that Mr. Cunningham's treatment regimen may include pegylated interferon. Which of the following is true regarding interferon in the general HCV-positive population?

   A. Male gender is a risk factor for interferon-induced depression.
   B. There is a cumulative 25% risk of interferon-induced depression.
   C. Pegylated interferon is contraindicated in patients with psychiatric history.
   D. Prophylaxis against interferon-induced depression is indicated regardless of baseline depressive symptoms.

Clinical Case 2

Mr. Phan is a 40-year-old man who emigrated from Southeast Asia 4 years ago. He is unaware of any medical problems and he has not seen a doctor in over 10 years. He has struggled with nightmares for "many years" associated with persistent feelings of anxiety. He recently qualified for the state assistance medical program and he is in your office today for his initial intake. Mr. Phan denies any personal history of injection drug use. He is employed part time as a cashier at a local grocery store. He is unaware of any family history of liver disease. On the basis of his emigration history, you consider him at high risk for chronic HBV infection.

1. Which of the following combination of tests indicates immunity from resolved HBV?[1]

   A. −HBsAg, −IgG anti-HBc, −anti-HBs.
   B. −HBsAg, +IgG anti-HBc, +anti-HBs.
   C. −HBsAg, −IgG anti-HBc, +anti-HBs.
   D. +HBsAg, +IgG anti-HBc, −anti-HBs, −IgM anti-HBc.

2. Which of the following is true regarding viral hepatitis?

   A. Fulminant hepatitis is a common form of HBV.
   B. 95% of HBV-infected adult patients develop chronic HBV.
   C. 75%–85% of HCV infections become chronic.
   D. HDV can only duplicate in the presence of coexisting HCV.

3. Which of the following infections are acquired primarily via fecal-oral route?

   A. HAV and HEV.
   B. HAV and HBV.
   C. HBV and HCV.
   D. HDV and HEV.

Clinical Case 3

Mr. Zollinger is a 38-year-old Army veteran with a history of bipolar I disorder who has been diagnosed with HCV. His bipolar I disorder is under control with lithium; he has not had a manic episode in over 4 years. He has continued to maintain his employment of 3 years at the Veterans Rehabilitation Center as a licensed vocational nurse. He made an appointment with a hepatologist and is now taking pegylated interferon. You have been made aware of Mr. Zollinger's medical development by the hepatologist.

1. Which of the following is evidence based regarding Mr. Zollinger's psychiatric disorder and upcoming HCV treatment?

   A. He is no more likely to experience higher rates of mania from interferon treatment than patients with no prior psychiatric diagnosis.
   B. He should not be treated with interferon-based treatment because it may induce manic symptoms.

---

[1]HBsAg = hepatitis B surface antigen; IgG anti-HBc = hepatitis B core antibody immunoglobulin G; Anti-HBs = hepatitis B surface antibody; IgM anti-HBc = hepatitis B core antibody immunoglobulin M.

C. His psychiatric disorder has been shown to negatively affect sustained viral response.
D. His rate of treatment completion is slower compared to nonpsychiatric HCV-positive patients.

CHAPTER 18

HIV/AIDS

Clinical Case 1

Mr. Williams, a 35-year-old single man, is back in your clinic 2 years after his last visit. He complains of excessive anxiety and worry that is consistent with his prior diagnosis of generalized anxiety disorder. He tells you that he lost his job 2 years ago. Since then, he had been incarcerated for several months following possession of drug paraphernalia. He admits to using intravenous methamphetamine and to trading sex with both men and women for drugs and alcohol. He has engaged in receptive anal intercourse with no barrier protection. He identifies as a heterosexual. He wants to get his anxiety disorder under control and stop using methamphetamines. As part of your comprehensive intake assessment, you decide to screen him for HIV. He was negative for HIV infection when you screened him 4 years ago. His screening test is now positive for HIV infection.

1. Which of the following is associated with better outcomes for this patient as it relates to his HIV infection?

   A. Male gender.
   B. Comorbid diagnosis of a mental health disorder.
   C. Diagnosis of HIV infection early in the disease course.
   D. HIV-targeted vaccination.

2. You have referred Mr. Williams to a primary care doctor. In the meantime, he continues to see you for ongoing comprehensive mental health care. He has no complaints and appears to be in fair physical health. Which of these tests could be useful in assessing the severity of his HIV infection?

A. Comprehensive metabolic panel.
B. CD4 cell count.
C. Hepatitis C virus antibody.
D. Urine toxicology.

3. Which of the following in Mr. Williams's history is a risk factor for HIV infection?

   A. Age.
   B. History of receptive anal intercourse without barrier protection.
   C. Prior diagnosis of generalized anxiety disorder.
   D. Marital status.

4. Which of the following behavioral interventions has the most evidence for effective reduction of HIV transmission?

   A. Provision of condoms to patients after every clinic visit.
   B. Male circumcision.
   C. Scheduling frequent visits.
   D. Single-session sexually transmitted disease risk reduction interventions.

Clinical Case 2

Ms. Ford, a 45-year-old divorced woman with history of HIV infection and bipolar I disorder, is following up with you after a 2-week hospitalization for a manic episode in the county psychiatric health facility. She was diagnosed with HIV infection 18 months ago but unfortunately has not been followed up for treatment. Her urine pregnancy test is negative.

1. In addition to promptly referring the patient to an infectious disease specialist for initiation of antiretroviral treatment, you check her CD4 count and HIV viral load. Which of the following levels of CD4 count should warrant consideration for prophylaxis against opportunistic infections?

   A. 1,000 cell/mm^3.
   B. 550 cell/mm^3.
   C. 300 cell/mm^3.
   D. 180 cell/mm^3.

2. You note that Ms. Ford's CD4 count is 150 cells/mm^3 and you discern that prophylaxis for *Pneumocystis jirovecii* pneumonia is indicated. Which of the following medications is appropriate?

   A. Penicillin.
   B. Trimethoprim/sulfamethoxazole (TMP-SMX).
   C. Azithromycin.
   D. Doxycycline.

3. You review Ms. Ford's discharge medications and note that she was discharged on carbamazepine. You are most worried about potential drug-drug interactions with which of the following?

   A. Indinavir.
   B. Ritonavir.
   C. Fluconazole.
   D. Efavirenz.

4. Which of the following minority populations shares the highest burden of HIV disease?

   A. Men who have sex with men.
   B. African American women.
   C. Latina women.
   D. Injection drug users.

Clinical Case 3

Mr. Butler is a 55-year-old man with history of hypertension and schizophrenia. His treatment course has been complicated by recurrent hospitalizations for acute decompensation, usually in the setting of medication nonadherence and methamphetamine intoxication. He was most recently discharged to a board and care facility for increased level of care.

1. According to a multisite prospective study in 2001, the prevalence of HIV infection among individuals with severe mental illness, compared to the general population, was found to be which of the following?

   A. Half the rate in the general population.
   B. The same rate as in the general population.
   C. Two times the rate in the general population.
   D. Greater than three times the rate in the general population.

2. You are reviewing Mr. Butler's medical records and note that he is linked with the university HIV treatment center, where he has been treated for over 2 years. You are concerned about overall adherence to his medications. Which of the following is true?

   A. HIV replicates quickly in its life cycle and quickly adjusts to any given antiviral medication if taken intermittently.
   B. HIV replicates slowly in its life cycle and develops resistance to antiviral medications if taken intermittently.
   C. HIV replicates slowly in its life cycle and has a low mutation rate.
   D. The course of HIV infection is not affected by inconsistent adherence to antiviral medications.

SECTION V

Oncological Disorders in the Psychiatric Patient Population

Section Editors:

Jaesu Han, M.D.

Lorin M. Scher, M.D.

Amy Nuismer, M.D.

With

Katerina Christiansen, M.D.

CHAPTER 19

Breast Cancer

Clinical Case 1

Ms. Alfonso is a 37-year-old premenopausal white woman with a diagnosis of generalized anxiety disorder who presents to her psychiatrist's office for a follow-up appointment. She has been taking fluoxetine 40 mg/day for several years and was doing well until recently. She has been particularly distressed since her 45-year-old sister was diagnosed with an infiltrating ductal carcinoma. Ms. Alfonso reports no other family members with a history of breast cancer and has been unable to sleep because she has been worrying about an achy, tender area of lumpy tissue felt in her right breast.

1. Which of the following would make you less suspicious for a primary cancer of the breast?

   A. Nipple discharge that is bloody in character.
   B. Dimpling skin changes with an inverted nipple.
   C. An area of mobile, ropelike tissue in the upper outer quadrant.
   D. A hard, fixed 2-cm mass with irregular borders.

2. Ms. Alfonso asks if smoking can cause her to develop breast cancer. Which are the most important risk factors for breast cancer?

   A. Family history of breast cancer and age.
   B. Age and gender.
   C. Early menarche and Caucasian race.
   D. History of proliferative breast tissue with atypia and gender.

3. Based on the American Cancer Society 2013 preventive guidelines, what is the best plan for Ms. Alfonso?

   A. Referral for a screening mammogram starting at age 40.
   B. Scheduling a clinical breast examination annually.

C. Clinician-based teaching and encouragement to do breast self-examinations monthly.
D. Having a breast magnetic resonance imaging (MRI) study starting at age 50.

Clinical Case 2

Mrs. Inah is a 50-year-old Russian woman with schizophrenia whose illness has been stabilized with clozapine for several years. She substitute teaches at a local high school and lives independently. Despite not having a primary care doctor, she rarely misses an appointment with you, her treating psychiatrist. She recently completed a screening mammogram at a mobile health clinic that came to her neighborhood. The mammogram results demonstrated a nonpalpable 5-cm mass in her left breast.

1. Which is the next most appropriate step in her management?

   A. Ultrasound-guided core needle biopsy.
   B. Surgical, open biopsy.
   C. Clinical follow-up and repeat imaging via MRI.
   D. Fine-needle aspiration of an axillary node.

2. Mrs. Inah is diagnosed with invasive breast cancer. Which of the following is not a consideration in the treatment?

   A. Axillary staging of disease.
   B. Tumor size.
   C. Human epidermal growth factor receptor 2 gene (*HER2*) status.
   D. Breast hormone analysis.

3. Mrs. Inah now faces chemotherapy. Which possible side effect or interaction between her psychotropic and chemotherapeutic agents should you, as her psychiatrist, consider?

   A. Blood dyscrasias leading to myelosuppression when used in combination with cytotoxic chemotherapeutic agents.
   B. Altered metabolism of oncological therapies and other pharmacokinetic interactions.
   C. QT_C prolongation when used in combination with antiemetic medications.
   D. All of the above.
   E. None of the above.

CHAPTER 20

Prostate Cancer

Clinical Case 1

Mr. Stewart, a 55-year-old white man, is a Vietnam veteran with a history of schizophrenia and tobacco abuse who presents for psychiatric follow-up. He does not have a primary care provider. During your visit, you discover he has been having nocturia and increased urinary frequency. Mr. Stewart is concerned because his friend with similar symptoms recently died of metastatic prostate cancer.

1. Which of the following is a risk factor for prostate cancer?

    A. Caucasian ethnicity.
    B. History of sexually transmitted infection.
    C. Exposure to Agent Orange.
    D. History of schizophrenia.

On further questioning, you discover that Mr. Stewart had a brother and uncle with prostate cancer diagnosed in their 60s. After careful discussion of the risks and benefits of prostate-specific antigen (PSA) screening, he elects to have his PSA level checked.

2. Which of the following is a true statement regarding prostate cancer screening?

    A. PSA testing may lead to early detection of prostate cancer.
    B. The majority of prostate cancers detected by screening will be fatal.

C. Treatment of early prostate cancer detected by PSA screening cannot cause harm to the patient.
D. It is always recommended to routinely offer PSA screening to average-risk individuals.

3. Mr. Stewart's PSA level returns at 10 ng/mL. What would be the best next step?

   A. Schedule a biopsy.
   B. Referral to urology.
   C. Start androgen deprivation therapy.
   D. Repeat a PSA screening in 1 year.

Clinical Case 2

Mr. Godfrey is an 85-year-old man with history of depression, anxiety, end-stage chronic obstructive pulmonary disease (COPD) (on home oxygen), and hypertension. He presents to your office for routine follow-up. While discussing his recent anxiety, he states that he recently read a story about a man with metastatic prostate cancer, and he is now convinced he should be checked for prostate cancer. He denies nocturia; change in urinary frequency, urgency, or hesitancy; or hematuria.

1. Which of the following aspects of Mr. Godfrey's history makes him more likely to be screened for prostate cancer?

   A. Hypertension.
   B. Depression.
   C. Anxiety.
   D. COPD.

2. After a long discussion with his physician, Mr. Godfrey insists on PSA screening. Which of the following is a reason *not* to screen for prostate cancer in this patient's case?

   A. His age.
   B. His end-stage COPD.
   C. The accrual of psychiatric illnesses due to overdiagnosis of low-risk cancers.
   D. All the above.
   E. None of the above.

3. Although many patients are very concerned about prostate cancer, which of the following is a true statement regarding the disease course?

   A. Prostate cancer is the most common malignancy diagnosed in men.
   B. Annual death rate from prostate cancer is very high.
   C. Roughly 50% of men will have occult prostate cancer at the time of their death.
   D. Men with prostate cancer confined to the organ at the time of diagnosis can expect a nearly 50% survival at 5 years.

CHAPTER 21

Lung Cancer

Clinical Case 1

Ms. Hodges is a 68-year-old woman who presents with a 3-month history of dry cough, blood-tinged sputum, and 10-lb unintentional weight loss. She denies fevers, chills, sore throat, chest pain, and abdominal pain. She has a past medical history of hypertension, type 2 diabetes, and chronic obstructive pulmonary disease (COPD). Her family history is significant for a brother who was recently diagnosed with lung cancer. She has a 25 pack-year history of smoking. Upon examination, her breath sounds are diminished with minimal expiratory wheezes. A chest X ray revealed a 4-cm mass in the left lower lobe.

1. Which aspect of her history puts Ms. Hodges at highest risk for developing lung cancer?

   A. Her gender.
   B. History of COPD.
   C. Smoking history.
   D. Family history of lung cancer.

2. You decide to refer your patient to a primary care physician for further follow-up. In the meantime, however, what is the next best step after chest X ray?

   A. Fine-needle biopsy.
   B. Computed tomography (CT) scan with contrast.
   C. Positron emission tomography (PET) scan.
   D. Sputum cytology.

3. Biopsy revealed a stage II non–small cell lung cancer (NSCLC). What would be the recommended treatment strategy for Ms. Hodges?

   A. Radiation therapy for palliative care.
   B. Chemotherapy and radiation therapy.
   C. Surgery and radiation therapy.
   D. Surgery, chemotherapy, and possibly radiation therapy.

Clinical Case 2

Mr. Devoe is a 55-year-old man with a history of depression, hypertension, and tobacco abuse who presents to your clinic for follow-up. He complains of occasional cough and denies fevers, dyspnea, chest pain, or unintentional weight loss. He says he has a 35 pack-year smoking history but has cut back to one pack per day. His vital signs today are as follows: blood pressure 180/82 mmHg, pulse 88 bpm, respiratory rate 17, and oxygen saturation 97%. Physical examination is unremarkable. Labs reveal a serum sodium level of 129 mEq/L and calcium level of 7.9 mEq/L.

1. Which of the following would be the best strategy for primary prevention of lung cancer in Mr. Devoe?

   A. Yearly chest X-ray.
   B. Smoking cessation.
   C. Yearly low-dose CT (LDCT) screening.
   D. Blood pressure control.

2. Because of Mr. Devoe's 35 pack-year smoking history and current smoking status, you recommend that he undergo LDCT screening. What is a potential disadvantage of LDCT surveillance?

   A. A significant rate of false-positive LDCT results.
   B. Further invasive procedures with inherent risks.
   C. Emotional stress due to suspicious lesions.
   D. All of the above.
   E. None of the above.

3. The LDCT scan demonstrates a 5-cm mass in Mr. Devoe's left upper lobe. You refer him to a pulmonologist, who performs a CT-guided biopsy, which reveals limited-stage small cell lung cancer (SCLC). Which of the following is true regarding SCLC?

A. SCLC accounts for the vast majority of lung cancers.
B. Limited-stage SCLC has a modest 5-year survival rate.
C. Extensive-stage SCLC has a high survival rate at 5 years.
D. Paraneoplastic syndromes are more common with NSCLC.

CHAPTER 22

Colorectal Cancer

Clinical Case 1

Mr. Wesley is a 55-year-old white man with schizophrenia who avoids going to see his primary care doctor because he believes the doctor dabbles in black magic. His body mass index (BMI) has remained at 42 for several years, and his favorite food is barbequed steak, which he eats daily. He drinks a six-pack of beer and smokes two packs of cigarettes per day. He expresses concern during his visit today about his stools, which have been alternating between "snakes and worms" for the past several months, and he has occasionally seen blood in his stool.

1. Which of the following does not increase Mr. Wesley's risk for colorectal cancer?

   A. Caucasian race.
   B. Male gender.
   C. Barbequed steak.
   D. Alcohol consumption.
   E. Obesity.

2. Mr. Wesley is not a candidate for colon cancer screening because of which of the following reasons?

   A. He presents with hematochezia.
   B. He has active symptoms of schizophrenia.
   C. He has average risk and is not yet age 60.
   D. He is not losing weight.

3. Mr. Wesley agrees to undergo diagnostic colonoscopy, and a 5-mm adenomatous polyp is found. What is the likelihood that an adenomatous polyp will evolve into an adenocarcinoma?

   A. <1%.
   B. <10%.
   C. 50%.
   D. >90%.

Clinical Case 2

Mrs. Darby is 50 years old and has a history of panic disorder with agoraphobia for which she no longer takes any medications. She is worried and anxious about the possibility of developing colorectal cancer. She denies any gastrointestinal symptoms, and her review of systems is negative. She is worried that screening can require multiple procedures.

1. Which screening option would allow Mrs. Darby to complete colorectal cancer screening and potential treatment in one procedure?

   A. Fecal occult blood testing.
   B. Colonoscopy.
   C. Flexible sigmoidoscopy.
   D. Fecal immunochemical testing.
   E. Computed tomographic colonography.

2. Mrs. Darby has been experiencing more panic attacks and engaging in avoidant behaviors as a result. In this patient with moderate symptoms, what would be the most appropriate next step for screening?

   A. Schedule a colonoscopy.
   B. Adjust the treatment for her panic disorder and reassess symptom control at her next visit before scheduling colorectal cancer screening.
   C. Order fecal occult blood testing.
   D. Defer screening until she is 60 years old, when she will be at higher risk for colorectal cancer.

3. Which of the following patients does *not* need referral to a specialist?

   A. A 54-year-old man with schizophrenia complaining of hematochezia for the past 3 months.
   B. A 58-year-old woman with bipolar I disorder who is asymptomatic but had an abnormal fecal immunochemical test.

C. A 36-year-old man with a 15-year history of inflammatory bowel disease.
D. A 44-year-old woman with schizoaffective disorder whose mother had colorectal cancer in her 80s.

CHAPTER 23

Cervical Cancer

Clinical Case 1

Ms. Ramos is a 23-year-old Latina woman with bipolar I disorder that is currently well controlled with lithium and carbamazepine. She is uncertain if she has ever had a Papanicolaou (Pap) smear but recalls receiving a human papilloma virus (HPV) vaccination when she was 19 years old. She has had multiple partners in the past 2 years. She does not endorse current symptoms. She has a levonorgestrel intrauterine device in place to prevent pregnancy.

1. What do current guidelines suggest for preventive cervical cancer screening for this patient?

   A. Cytology every 3 years.
   B. Cytology annually.
   C. Cytology every 5 years and HPV cotesting.
   D. She no longer needs screening because she has been vaccinated for HPV.

2. Ms. Ramos expresses misconceptions regarding screening and states that she feels uncomfortable around new health care providers. Which intervention is the most appropriate in her case?

   A. Bring screening visits into the mental health center.
   B. Provide education around screening with accurate information.
   C. Provide a personal recommendation for a primary care physician.
   D. Inquire into the reasons for her discomfort and address her concerns.
   E. All of the above.

3. Ms. Ramos eventually agrees to have a Pap smear. Results reveal atypical squamous cells of undetermined significance (ASCUS) and negative HPV on reflex testing. What is the next step in management?

   A. Hysterectomy.
   B. Colposcopy.
   C. Repeat cytology in 12 months.
   D. Repeat cytology in 3 years.

Clinical Case 2

Mrs. Evans is a 50-year-old white woman with borderline personality disorder who has been working with you as her treating psychiatrist as well as a psychotherapist for several years. She reluctantly informs you of a traumatic, sexually abusive encounter, which makes it very difficult for her to tolerate pelvic examinations despite a good working relationship with her primary care physician.

1. Mrs. Evans's primary care physician calls you to discuss alternatives because the patient continues to decline a pelvic examination. Which of the following is the best option for this patient?

   A. HPV testing alone.
   B. Stop offering pelvic examinations.
   C. Peer education and support groups.
   D. Offer an examination under anesthesia.

2. Mrs. Evans eventually agrees to cervical cancer screening but "only the bare minimum frequency." Which screening schedule would be the most appropriate for this patient?

   A. Cytology every 3 years.
   B. Cytology annually.
   C. Cytology every 5 years with HPV cotesting.
   D. Cytology every 10 years with HPV cotesting.

3. Mrs. Evans agrees to a Pap smear. The results arrive 3 weeks later and demonstrate adenoma in situ. What is the next best step in her management?

   A. Serial colposcopy and cytology.
   B. Ablation.
   C. Hysterectomy.
   D. Excision and close follow-up.

CHAPTER 24

Skin Cancers

Clinical Case 1

Ms. Morris is a 49-year-old white woman with schizophrenia and traumatic brain injury after a motor vehicle accident 6 years ago. She has difficulty learning and, despite counseling, never remembers to wear sunscreen. She has red hair and a fair complexion. She wants to have a tan and asks if it is safe to go to an ultraviolet (UV) light tanning salon.

1. This patient should be encouraged to do which of the following to decrease her risk of developing a skin malignancy?

   A. Wear sunscreen with an SPF of 30 or more.
   B. Avoid tanning beds.
   C. Avoid excessive sun exposure.
   D. All of the above.
   E. None of the above.

2. Ms. Morris shows you a 1-cm papule on the back of her left hand. It is pearly and translucent with telangiectasias. What is the most likely diagnosis?

   A. Nodular basal cell carcinoma.
   B. Squamous cell carcinoma.
   C. Actinic keratosis.
   D. Superficial spreading melanoma.

3. Which of the following accurately describes the natural history of the type of lesion that Ms. Morris has?

   A. It is fast growing.
   B. Metastasis is common.
   C. It may result in significant tissue destruction and disfigurement if left untreated.
   D. It commonly develops from a preexisting actinic keratosis lesion.

Clinical Case 2

Mrs. Riley is a 66-year-old woman with obsessive-compulsive disorder who presents to your office with a 7-mm lesion of her left upper thigh. She tells you that it began as a mole but it has enlarged over the past 2 months. She reports that recently the borders have become asymmetrical and multicolored (including black, brown, and dark purple).

1. What is the most likely diagnosis?

   A. Nodular basal cell carcinoma.
   B. Squamous cell carcinoma.
   C. Actinic keratosis.
   D. Superficial spreading melanoma.

2. What is the next step in management for Mrs. Riley's diagnosis?

   A. Incisional biopsy.
   B. Excisional biopsy.
   C. Cryotherapy.
   D. Topical 5-fluorouracil.
   E. Photodynamic therapy.

3. Mrs. Riley is eventually started on interferon alfa-2b. Close monitoring for which of the following neuropsychiatric symptoms is recommended?

   A. Severe mania or depression.
   B. Memory loss.
   C. Auditory hallucinations.
   D. Leaden paralysis.

SECTION VI

Geriatric Preventive Care

Section Editors:

Jaesu Han, M.D.

Lorin M. Scher, M.D.

Erica Heiman, M.D.

With

Aleea Maye, M.D.

Steven R. Chan, M.D., M.B.A.

CHAPTER 25

Geriatric Preventive Care

Clinical Case 1

Mr. Allen, an 82-year-old white man with recurrent major depressive disorder and a past suicide attempt, slowly walks into your clinic with a staggering gait. He is unable to rise from his chair without the use of his upper arms. He is currently taking diltiazem for congestive heart failure and rate control of his atrial fibrillation, as well as metoprolol, dabigatran, and sertraline. Several bruises appear on his skin. He lives on the second story of his three-story house. He lives alone, his mood has been stable for the last 3 years, and his score on the Montreal Cognitive Assessment (MoCA) is 28/30.

1. Which is the most likely diagnosis for Mr. Allen?

   A. Iatrogenic fall.
   B. Muscular dystrophy.
   C. Elder abuse.
   D. Parkinson's dementia.

2. Mr. Allen has a heart rate of 55 and is euvolemic. What is the next best step in the management of his condition?

   A. Use of a cardiac pacemaker.
   B. Reduction of diltiazem.
   C. Reduction of sertraline.
   D. Use of compression stockings.

3. Performing the next step in management as listed in the previous question is an example of which type of prevention?

   A. Primary prevention.
   B. Secondary prevention.
   C. Tertiary prevention.
   D. Quaternary prevention.

Clinical Case 2

Mr. Robinson, an 86-year-old black man with bipolar disorder and cataracts, lives in an isolated rural house and relies on his caregiver for transport. The patient complains of decreased energy and depressed mood. He has lost approximately 5% of his baseline body weight over the last half year. He has missed 50% of his appointments, and his most recent prescriptions for lithium and citalopram have not been filled for 2 months. The patient complains of constantly being hungry.

1. What is the most common cause of involuntary weight loss in older adults?

   A. SSRI side effect.
   B. Depression.
   C. Dysphagia.
   D. Cancer.

2. For which of the following patients should routine colon cancer screening be considered?

   A. A patient who is 75 years old with no history.
   B. A patient who is 85 years old with a history of colon cancer.
   C. A patient who is 85 years old with a history of colon cancer.
   D. A patient who is 95 years old without a history of colon cancer.

3. What is an important next step in the management of Mr. Robinson's condition?

   A. Refer him to a primary care provider for prostate-specific antigen (PSA) screening and digital rectal examination.
   B. Refill medications and add mirtazapine.
   C. Ask, "Have your belongings been taken from you without your permission?"
   D. Ask, "Do you feel dissatisfied with the way your body looks?"

Clinical Case 3

Ms. Scott, a 66-year-old woman with diabetes, generalized anxiety disorder, and alcohol use disorder in sustained full remission, presents to your clinic in autumn. She updated her vaccinations last year but missed her tetanus vaccine. She is unsure if she has ever received a combined tetanus, diphtheria, pertussis (Tdap) vaccination, and is concerned that her memory is "not as good as it used to be."

1. What vaccinations are indicated for Ms. Scott?

   A. Live attenuated intranasal influenza and Tdap.
   B. Live attenuated intranasal influenza and tetanus and diphtheria vaccine (Td).
   C. Inactivated intramuscular influenza and Tdap.
   D. Inactivated intradermal influenza and Td.

2. Which supplements have been found to be associated with a decreased risk of all-cause dementia?

   A. Vitamin B_{12} and folic acid.
   B. Vitamins C and E.
   C. Ginkgo biloba.
   D. Omega-3 fatty acid.

3. Ms. Scott smells of cigarette smoke. She complains of seeing blind spots and needing to use a magnifying glass. She also complains that straight lines on a page appear distorted. What would you recommend for this patient?

   A. Taking vitamins C and E.
   B. Having cataract removal surgery.
   C. None are indicated, as supplements are not associated with preventing glaucoma.
   D. None are indicated for primary prevention.

Clinical Case 4

Mr. Jackson is an 80-year-old man with a history of coronary artery disease following a coronary artery bypass graft 10 years ago, type 2 diabetes, hypertension, macular degeneration, benign prostatic hypertrophy, generalized anxiety disorder, and depression. He presents to your clinic with a caregiver to follow up on his anxiety. His caregiver mentions that the patient had two falls last week as he was getting out of bed to go to the bathroom at night. The patient would rather discuss how his anxiety has worsened over the past few weeks, and he would like more medication to help him during this difficult time.

1. Initial approaches toward fall reduction for this patient should include which of the following?

   A. Complete medication reconciliation.
   B. Discontinuation of blood pressure medications.
   C. Discontinuation of any blood thinners, including aspirin.
   D. Referral to physical therapy.

2. Which of the following best predicts increased risk of falls in patients such as Mr. Jackson?

   A. Worsening symptoms of anxiety.
   B. History of high blood pressure.
   C. Deficits in 5-minute object recall.
   D. Inability to stand unassisted, walk 10 feet, and then return to seated position within 10 seconds.

3. Mr. Jackson additionally reports to you that he does not have a clear memory of his falls. He remembers standing up, feeling lightheaded, experiencing palpitations, and then being on the floor afterward. The fall itself is "a blur." Given this history, which of the following is most likely?

   A. Peripheral neuropathy.
   B. Visual deficits.
   C. Elder abuse.
   D. Orthostatic syncope.

Clinical Case 5

Ms. Mason is an 80-year-old woman with a history of vascular dementia, chronic obstructive pulmonary disease, hypertension, and depression. She is dependent on her daughter for instrumental activities of daily living as well as bathing and dressing. She is brought to your clinic to follow up on her depression. Her daughter, who accompanies her to the visit, provides her mother's history and reports being worried because her mother has recently seemed "detached," not participating at her usual Tuesday evening bingo games or in family discussions at dinner.

1. Which of the following tests might you consider as you approach the changes in Ms. Mason's behavior?

    A. A hearing test.
    B. Vision testing.
    C. Mini-Mental State Examination (MMSE), MoCA, or other cognitive test.
    D. All of the above.

2. The neurological examination shows diminished acuity of peripheral vision in both eyes. Ms. Mason has no orbital pain. What is her most likely diagnosis?

    A. Diabetic retinopathy.
    B. Macular degeneration.
    C. Open-angle glaucoma.
    D. Acoustic neuroma.

3. Which of the following preventive health options is most appropriate for Ms. Mason at this time?

    A. Referral for a colonoscopy.
    B. Mammography.
    C. Zoster (shingles) vaccine.
    D. Meningococcal vaccine.

Clinical Case 6

Mr. Moore is a 76-year-old physician. Although he has had to cut back his working hours because of arthritic pain and "slowing down," he continues to practice, and his work is well appreciated by his colleagues and patients. He lives in a single-story apartment with his wife of 50 years and their dog. He continues to be physically active and walk his dog twice daily. He manages his own finances and medications. Current medications are aspirin 81 mg/day, simvastatin (to treat dyslipidemia), amlodipine (to treat hypertension), citalopram (to treat depression), and omeprazole (to treat gastritis).

1. Mr. Moore's last colonoscopy was 10 years ago, and the results were normal. He requests that you order a new colonoscopy for him. Which of the following is the most appropriate clinical approach?

A. A colonoscopy would be inappropriate for a patient of his age; no colorectal cancer screening should be done.
B. He can be screened, but a less invasive modality such as fecal immunochemical testing or flexible sigmoidoscopy is more appropriate than colonoscopy.
C. Given his excellent functional status, it is appropriate to send the patient for colonoscopy.
D. It is inappropriate to screen him again because the likelihood that a new malignant lesion or premalignant lesions have appeared in the last 10 years is very low.

2. Regarding global assessment of function, which elderly group does Mr. Moore fit into?

A. Independent function, with or without chronic disease and with life expectancy of more than 5 years.
B. Dependent function, with multiple chronic morbidities and life expectancy of 2–5 years.
C. Nearing the end of life, with life expectancy of less than 2 years.
D. Pseudo-elderly, with life expectancy of more than 20 years.

3. Mr. Moore has no complaints at today's visit. His mood is currently good, but he has a history of three episodes of major depressive disorder, the last of which occurred 4 years ago. His blood pressure is at target range, and he has had no chest pain, abdominal pain, or gastroesophageal reflux disorder (GERD) symptoms in the last 6 months. What is another action you could consider at today's visit?

A. Ordering a PSA level for prostate cancer screening.
B. Administering an MMSE for dementia screening.
C. Discontinuing simvastatin because he has no cardiac history or chest pain.
D. Discontinuing omeprazole because of no evidence of active GERD.

Clinical Case 7

Ms. Reiter is an 86-year-old woman with a history of depression, mild cognitive impairment, hypertension, and seasonal allergies. The patient lives with her daughter and son-in-law. Her daughter accompanies her to the clinic today. Her daughter reports that the patient is doing "fine" but that the patient's son-in-law, who stays with Ms. Reiter when the daughter is at work, has more information on the patient's day-to-day activities. The patient also claims that she is "fine," but you notice that she does not maintain eye contact and appears distressed. She has lost 15 lbs since her last visit with you 3 months ago.

1. You are concerned about elder abuse. Which of the following is the most appropriate action at this time?

   A. Contact adult protective services immediately.
   B. Kindly ask the patient's daughter to step out of the room, and then ask the patient, "Do you feel uncomfortable with anyone who is taking care of you?"
   C. Include this suspicion in your chart note and make sure to follow up at the next visit.
   D. Increase the patient's citalopram dose because this presentation may represent worsening depression.

2. Which of the following is the prevalence of elder abuse in the community, per best estimates?

   A. <1%.
   B. 2%–10%.
   C. 10%–30%.
   D. 25%–50%.

3. Which of the following is a risk factor for elder mistreatment?

   A. Depression and cognitive impairment.
   B. Female gender.
   C. Living with family members.
   D. Hypertension.

Clinical Case 8

Mrs. Sable is a 70-year-old woman with a history of major depression, anxiety, chronic pain, diabetes, chronic kidney disease, coronary artery disease, and hypertension. She comes to the clinic with her son for follow-up of worsening anxiety. She lives with her son and is able to perform all activities of daily living independently with the exception of using a walker for gait stability. She takes all medications as prescribed but has not seen a primary care physician in more than 10 years and has no history of abnormal pap smears. While her history is being gathered, it is uncovered that Mrs. Sable has had an unintentional weight loss of 20 lbs in the past 6 months.

1. What is the next best step in further evaluating Mrs. Sable's weight loss?

   A. Obtain a complete review of systems.
   B. Inform patient of the need for a positron emission tomography (PET) scan to rule out cancer.
   C. Obtain medication reconciliation.
   D. Answers A and C.

2. Upon further questioning, you find that Mrs. Sable has been experiencing the following symptoms over the past few weeks: intermittent palpitations, stomach upset, and loose stools. Current medications include clonazepam, sertraline, insulin, hydrocodone/acetaminophen, lisinopril, metoprolol, simvastatin, and aspirin. What is the most likely cause of Mrs. Sable's weight loss?

   A. Sertraline.
   B. Malignancy.
   C. Hyperthyroidism.
   D. Anorexia of old age.

3. What cancer screening test(s) would be appropriate to recommend at this time?

   A. Colonoscopy.
   B. Mammography.
   C. Papanicolaou smear.
   D. Colonoscopy and mammography.

Clinical Case 9

Mr. Paliski is a 79-year-old wheelchair-bound black man with a history of cerebrovascular accident with residual right-sided weakness, bipolar affective disorder, mild dementia, hypertension, heart failure, and coronary artery disease. He lives with his son and daughter-in-law and their four young children. He comes to the clinic with his daughter-in-law to follow up on his bipolar affective disorder. Of note, Mr. Paliski typically has good hygiene; however, during this clinical encounter, he appears far more disheveled and engages minimally in the interview. His current medications include valproate, aspirin, carvedilol, furosemide, lisinopril, and simvastatin.

1. What medical testing is appropriate in this patient with worsening cognitive function?

   A. Thyroid-stimulating hormone (TSH) test.
   B. Lipid panel.

C. Hemoglobin A_{1c}.
D. Basal metabolic panel.

The patient's daughter-in-law reports giving Mr. Paliski some of her own lorazepam intermittently over the past few months to help with sleep, and more frequently over the past few weeks when he has become more agitated. His vital signs are within normal limits. Further review of symptoms is noncontributory. Depressive symptoms have remained unchanged in severity per history obtained from the patient and family. The patient refuses to cooperative with the MMSE or MoCA.

2. Which of the following would be the best action to address the patient's worsening agitation?

   A. Recommend that the daughter-in-law stop giving lorazepam to the patient.
   B. Recommend addition of quetiapine as needed for agitation.
   C. Prescribe lorazepam as needed for agitation, and educate the daughter-in-law on safe practices for as-needed use of lorazepam.
   D. Do not make medication changes and instead suggest behavioral plans for the daughter-in-law to use as needed.

3. What would be the appropriate preventive care measures for Mr. Paliski at this time, taking into account that his last pneumococcal and zoster vaccines were administered 13 years ago, his last Tdap vaccine 8 years age, and his last flu vaccine 1 year ago during the previous flu season?

   A. Recommend that the patient obtain one more dose of pneumococcal and Td vaccines.
   B. Recommend that the patient obtain an influenza vaccine.
   C. Recommend that the patient obtain a colonoscopy.
   D. Recommend addition of omega-3 fatty acids to the patient's diet.

Clinical Case 10

Mr. Zima is a 69-year-old man with a history of moderate to severe recurrent major depressive disorder, diabetes, hypertension, hyperlipidemia, coronary artery disease, and recent diagnosis of metastatic pancreatic cancer 3 months prior. He is currently undergoing palliative chemotherapy and radiation treatments. Given the poor prognosis for pancreatic cancer, he recently changed his code status to "do not resuscitate." He comes to the clinic with complaints of worsening depression. Significant findings on review of systems include acute-on-chronic pain, nausea and vomiting, and increased frequency of falls within the last few months. Current medications include sertraline, insulin, metoprolol, aspirin, simvastatin, and morphine.

1. What is the best line of inquiry to investigate the patient's increased falls?

   A. Evaluate for associated symptoms connected to falls.
   B. Discuss location and activities associated with the fall.
   C. Evaluate for sensory impairment including neurological screening for neuropathy and vision and hearing testing.
   D. All of the above.

2. Upon further inquiry, Mr. Zima reports that before his falls, he has experienced palpitations and chest pain followed by brief loss of consciousness. No gait abnormalities are detected during the examination, and his Timed Get Up and Go test result is within normal limits. What is the next best step in evaluation and management of falls for this patient?

   A. Send the patient to a cardiologist to evaluate the need for an implantable cardiac device.
   B. Discuss with the patient the likely diagnosis of cardiac arrhythmia and the risks and benefits of treatment versus no treatment.
   C. Recommend discontinuation of morphine because this medication is the likely cause.
   D. Recommend discontinuation of aspirin given the increased risk of bleeding in the setting of recurrent falls.

3. Mr. Zima's last colonoscopy was more than 10 years ago. He has had all recommended vaccinations. What preventive care measure is indicated for this patient?

   A. Offer him a PSA screening for prostate cancer.
   B. Recommend colon cancer screening with colonoscopy.
   C. Recommend vision and hearing screenings.
   D. Consider discussion regarding discontinuing simvastatin.

Clinical Case 11

Ms. Quan is a 66-year-old Chinese American woman who immigrated to the United States from Indonesia in 1998. She has a history of severe recurrent depression with anxious features and is currently taking aripiprazole and escitalopram. She asks you today about screening for low bone density. She saw an advertisement on television and thinks she may need this screening.

1. What action, if any, is appropriate to assess bone density and the possibility of fractures?

   A. Order dual-energy X-ray absorptiometry (DEXA), and use the composite L2–L4 T-score.
   B. Order DEXA and use the lowest two T-scores.
   C. Order a spinal computed tomography (CT) scan to evaluate bone density.
   D. Provide reassurance; there is no appropriate testing at this time.

2. Which medication(s) in the patient's regimen may put her at risk of osteoporosis?

   A. Escitalopram.
   B. Aripiprazole.
   C. Answers A and B.
   D. None of the above.

3. On follow-up, Ms. Quan returns for her appointment but has not completed the testing you have ordered. She has a history of missed clinic appointments. What is the next best step in the management of this patient?

   A. Ask questions from the Cultural Formulation Interview, including "What troubles you most about your problem?"
   B. Discharge the patient from your clinic, because her erratic behavior has made appropriate therapy too difficult.
   C. Order alendronate as empirical therapy for osteoporosis.
   D. Report the patient to adult protective services because elder abuse is clearly happening.

Clinical Case 12

Mrs. Sallie is a 68-year-old white woman with a history of mild cognitive impairment, hypertension, hyperlipidemia, and depression. She comes to your clinic for follow-up on her clinical depression. During the evaluation she mentions that her mother suffered from Alzheimer's dementia, and Mrs. Sallie would like to know if there are any natural substances she can use to help prevent her from progressing to dementia. She brings this up after watching an ad for ginkgo biloba supplements that help with memory and would like to know whether this is an appropriate supplement to take to preserve her memory.

1. How do you respond to the patient's inquiry regarding ginkgo biloba?

   A. Encourage her to start taking ginkgo biloba supplements because evidence has shown that it is helpful for preventing cognitive decline.
   B. Encourage her to consider omega-3 fatty acids because evidence has shown that these are helpful for slowing cognitive decline.
   C. Encourage her to consider increasing exercise and vegetables in her diet because evidence suggests that these measures may be helpful in slowing cognitive decline.
   D. Inform the patient that no interventions have been proven to prevent and slow cognitive decline.

2. Mrs. Sallie would like to know if there are any other interventions that may help with slowing or preventing further cognitive decline. How do you respond?

   A. Inform the patient that she should consider adding vitamins E and C.
   B. Inform the patient that she should consider folic acid and vitamin B_6.
   C. Inform the patient that the next best option would be to undergo cognitive training to improve current cognitive functioning.
   D. Advise the patient to consider starting vitamin B_{12} supplements.

3. What would be the appropriate label for the type of intervention encouraged in the above question?

   A. Primary prevention.
   B. Secondary prevention.
   C. Tertiary prevention.
   D. None of the above.

SECTION VII

Child and Adolescent Preventive Care

Section Editor:

Glen L. Xiong, M.D.

Matthew Gibson, M.D.

With

Danielle Alexander, M.D.

CHAPTER 26

Child and Adolescent Preventive Care

Clinical Case 1

Mr. Taylor is a 24-year-old male with obsessive-compulsive personality disorder and type 1 diabetes. He is expecting his first child soon. Mr. Taylor's brother was diagnosed with attention-deficit/hyperactivity disorder (ADHD) at age 9. Mr. Taylor is concerned about his child developing ADHD too.

1. You advise Mr. Taylor that which of the following might decrease his child's risk of developing ADHD?

   A. Avoiding prenatal tobacco exposure.
   B. Avoiding prenatal lead exposure.
   C. Reducing psychosocial stressors.
   D. Answers A and C.
   E. All of the above.

2. Which of the following regarding the genetic basis of ADHD is true?

   A. ADHD is not a hereditary illness.
   B. Genetic predisposition to ADHD is less significant than environmental influences.
   C. Twin studies suggest that heritability of ADHD is very strong.
   D. Possessing any single gene associated with ADHD will likely lead to the illness.

3. ADHD affects approximately what percentage of adolescents ages 13–18 years?

   A. <1%.
   B. 1%–3%.
   C. 4%–6%.
   D. 7%–9%.

Clinical Case 2

Julia is a 7-year-old female referred by her primary care physician for poor sociability. Her father reports that she is having difficulty adjusting to school. Julia is the youngest of three children. Her birth history is unremarkable. Her developmental history is significant for delayed speech development. She is currently being treated for asthma and eczema.

1. As part of a complete history, which of the following details is important to obtain about Julia?

   A. Maternal exposure to the antiepileptic drug valproate.
   B. Maternal gestational diabetes.
   C. Paternal pack-year smoking history.
   D. Secondhand smoke exposure.
   E. Vaccination history.

2. Julia is diagnosed with ASD. Her father asks how he can decrease the risk that his next child will develop the illness. Which of the following should you recommend?

   A. No recommendation, because ASD is not a heritable illness.
   B. Daily maternal prenatal vitamins.
   C. Participation in first-trimester screening programs.
   D. Attendance at third-trimester prenatal care appointments.

3. What does the American College of Obstetricians and Gynecologists recommend for folic acid supplementation of reproductive-age women?

   A. 800 μg/day.
   B. 400 μg/day.
   C. 200 μg/day.
   D. 4.0 mg/day.
   E. 2.0 mg/day.

Clinical Case 3

Lucas is an 11-year-old male who is brought into the pediatrician's office by his maternal grandmother for insomnia. His father was recently arrested for molestation. Lucas experiences nightmares but is reluctant to provide details.

1. After thorough evaluation, you diagnose Lucas with posttraumatic stress disorder (PTSD). What is the best initial therapeutic intervention?

   A. Cognitive-behavioral therapy (CBT).
   B. Risperidone.
   C. Propranolol.
   D. Dyadic caregiver-child intervention.

2. Which of the following statements regarding propranolol is accurate?

   A. Propranolol has demonstrated efficacy for primary prevention of PTSD in adults.
   B. Propranolol may prevent the onset of PTSD by modification of the parasympathetic nervous system.
   C. In pediatric studies, propranolol has not been observed to be effective in PTSD prevention.
   D. Propranolol is one of many medications under investigation to prevent PTSD in children.

3. Given the diagnosis of PTSD, which of the following is Lucas most at risk for?

   A. Weight gain.
   B. Substance use disorder.
   C. Heart arrhythmia.
   D. Essential hypertension

Clinical Case 4

Daniel is an 8-year-old black male with ASD and prominent irritability who presents for a psychiatric follow-up. He has regular checkups with his pediatrician and no known medical problems. His family psychiatric and medical history is unremarkable. He is not currently taking any medications.

1. Which of the following measures should the treating psychiatrist monitor at routine intervals for this patient?

A. Heart rate and blood pressure.
B. Body mass index (BMI) percentile.
C. Waist circumference.
D. Lipid profile and fasting blood glucose.

2. The psychiatrist decides to add aripiprazole for treatment of irritability. Daniel's lipid profile, blood pressure, waist circumference, weight, and BMI are within normal limits for his age and sex. Baseline measures of what else should be obtained?

   A. Fasting blood sugar or glycosylated hemoglobin (HbA_{1c}).
   B. Electrocardiogram.
   C. Basal metabolic rate.
   D. Thyroid-stimulating hormone.

3. How often should the psychiatrist monitor this child's waist circumference, weight, and BMI?

   A. Every 6 months.
   B. Every 12 months.
   C. In 3 months, then every 6 months.
   D. At each visit.

Clinical Case 5

Sophia is a 15-year-old white female who presents for an initial outpatient psychiatric intake appointment. She was hospitalized 4 weeks ago for a first episode of acute mania and diagnosed with bipolar I disorder. Her symptoms were stabilized with the use of olanzapine, and she was discharged on this medication. The recorded BMI from her hospitalization was in the 77th percentile for her age and sex, but no labwork was done during her admission.

1. In addition to obtaining the appropriate baseline measurements for metabolic monitoring, which of the following is an appropriate intervention to implement at this point?

   A. Refer patient to a dietician to initiate a monitored dietary plan which induces a calorie deficit of approximately 500 calories per week.
   B. Encourage the consumption of a diet that is low in fast food, sodas, and added sugar.
   C. Initiate metformin 250 mg bid with meals.
   D. Encourage the consumption of a diet that includes a fruit drink with most meals.

2. Which statement represents the best advice for Sophia regarding physical activity?

   A. Group activities and team-based sports are encouraged above solitary activities.
   B. She should accumulate 150 minutes of exercise over the course of the week.
   C. Sedentary activities, such as playing video games, do not need to be limited as long as they are balanced with at least 30 minutes of exercise in the same day.
   D. Vigorous physical activity should be performed every other day, with a day of rest in between for recovery.

3. Which of the following should prompt urgent alert to Sophia's primary care provider for development of an individualized lifestyle modification treatment plan?

   A. BMI of 22.
   B. A 5% weight gain since starting olanzapine.
   C. Family history of myocardial infarction in multiple first-degree relatives.
   D. BMI in the 90th percentile for age and sex.

Clinical Case 6

Carl is a 17-year-old Filipino male with schizophrenia who presents for psychiatric follow-up. He has undergone multiple medication trials before achieving remission of his psychotic symptoms with a high dose of quetiapine. Three months ago his waist circumference was markedly elevated, and his BMI was in the 95th percentile for his height and weight. His parents have been helping him to carefully follow the balanced diet and exercise plan recommended by his primary care provider. Nevertheless, Carl's BMI is now in the 98th percentile, and his lipid profile is now remarkable for moderate elevation of triglycerides.

1. Which of the following has been shown to be most effective for weight loss in patients like Carl?

   A. Initiation and rapid titration of metformin.
   B. Strict adherence to an exercise regimen.
   C. Decrease in the dose of antipsychotic.
   D. Decrease in overall calorie intake.
   E. Initiation of a low dose of long-acting insulin.

2. Which of the following has evidence to support its use in attenuating or reversing weight gain related to SGA use in adolescents who are severely affected and resistant to lifestyle modification?

   A. Glyburide.
   B. Topiramate.
   C. Valproate.
   D. Phentermine.
   E. Lorcaserin.

3. Carl's psychiatrist decides to start metformin as an adjunctive means of weight control. What side effects should she warn Carl and his parents about?

   A. Abdominal cramping.
   B. Shortness of breath.
   C. Paresthesias.
   D. Nightmares.
   E. Palpitations.

Clinical Case 7

Brayden is a 14-year-old white male who is brought in by his mother for initial psychiatric evaluation because of "disruptive behavior" and smoking in the house. There is no known family history of psychiatric illness.

1. Which of the following statements most accurately reflects the relationship between early childhood adversity and subsequent risk of mental illness?

   A. Sexual abuse in childhood, but not physical abuse, has been associated with increased risk of developing a psychiatric disorder later in life.
   B. People who experienced a single traumatic event in their childhoods are at greater risk of developing mental illness than those who experienced multiple adversities.
   C. Approximately half of childhood-onset psychiatric disorders can be linked to childhood adversity.
   D. There is an association between early childhood adversity and the onset of mental illness in childhood, but not in adulthood.

2. Which represents the best approach to screening Brayden for early childhood adversity?

A. Ask him open-ended questions such as, "Were you traumatized in any way as a child?"
B. Establish rapport and wait for him to be comfortable enough to bring up any possible history of childhood trauma on his own.
C. Identify and screen for the form of adversity that is most likely to have affected him (e.g., physical abuse).
D. Systematically screen for multiple potential types of childhood adversity and for symptoms associated with those events.

3. The psychiatrist learns that Brayden was sexually abused as a child. Which of the following statements is most accurate regarding child abuse prevention programs?

   A. These programs have been proven to decrease the incidence of psychiatric disorders.
   B. They generally target older children who have been victims of abuse in the past.
   C. They tend to measure outcomes based on subsequent rates of abuse.
   D. The majority of these programs are held in juvenile detention facilities.

Clinical Case 8

Gabriela is a 15-year-old Hispanic female with major depressive disorder and generalized anxiety disorder who presents for psychiatric follow-up. She has a history of one suicide attempt, approximately 2 years ago, and of having been sexually trafficked in her early teens. She is making friends and good grades at her new high school, which was in the news last week for a cheerleader who committed suicide. She is not taking any medications.

1. How often should Gabriela be screened for suicidal ideation?

   A. At every visit.
   B. If symptoms of anxiety worsen.
   C. If a friend or classmate recently committed suicide.
   D. There is no need for routine screening.

2. Which factor uniquely amplifies risk of suicide in children and adolescents as opposed to adults?

   A. Previous history of suicide attempts.
   B. Comorbid depression and anxiety.
   C. Peer who committed suicide.

D. History of physical or sexual abuse.
E. Command auditory hallucinations.

3. Use of selective serotonin reuptake inhibitors (SSRIs) has been associated with treatment-emergent suicidality in pediatric patients. In the treatment of which disorder is this effect most pronounced?

   A. Major depressive disorder.
   B. Generalized anxiety disorder.
   C. Anxiety disorder not otherwise specified (other specified or unspecified anxiety disorder).
   D. Obsessive-compulsive disorder.
   E. Autism spectrum disorder.

Clinical Case 9

Thien is a 17-year-old Vietnamese female with obsessive-compulsive disorder who presents for psychiatric follow-up. Her condition is well controlled on a moderate dose of imipramine. She is now doing well in school, although before she engaged in treatment, she had significant behavior problems at school. She has been in a stable relationship for 6 months and denies suicidal ideation. She has no history of being abused.

1. Which factor increases Thien's risk for substance misuse over that of other adolescents?

   A. Diagnosis of obsessive-compulsive disorder.
   B. Female sex.
   C. Use of a tricyclic antidepressant.
   D. Being in a relationship.
   E. History of behavioral problems.

2. Which of the following is *not* one of the CRAFFT questions for substance abuse screening?

   A. Have you ever gotten into TROUBLE while you were using alcohol or drugs?
   B. Do you ever FORGET things you did while using alcohol or drugs?
   C. Have you ever felt you needed to CUT down on your alcohol or drug use?
   D. Do your family or FRIENDS ever tell you that you should cut down on drinking or drug use?
   E. Do you ever use alcohol or drugs while you are ALONE?

3. Which statement regarding the CRAFFT substance abuse screening questionnaire is accurate?

   A. A single positive response is a normal finding, which should not prompt further evaluation.
   B. Five or more positive responses are sufficient for the diagnosis of a substance use disorder.
   C. The instrument has been validated for individuals ages 12–30 years.
   D. Two or more positive responses suggest a significant substance use problem.

Clinical Case 10

Anna is a 12-year-old Ukrainian female with obsessive-compulsive disorder who presents for psychiatric follow-up. Her medical history is notable for asthma. She was recently seen by her pediatrician, who recommended several immunizations. Her mother refused all immunizations at that time because "the flu shot last year gave her the flu" and due to concern over articles she has read on the Internet linking vaccines and autism.

1. What is the most accurate statement regarding pediatric immunoprophylaxis?

   A. Vaccine recommendations in the United States have remained consistent over the past decade.
   B. Physicians are advised to consult the vaccine guidelines published in 2008 by the American Academy of Pediatrics.
   C. Two influenza vaccines are available for pediatric patients: the trivalent inactivated influenza vaccine and the live attenuated influenza vaccine.
   D. Parental beliefs about immunization risks are rarely altered by physician counseling.

2. Which of the following statements best reflects current vaccine recommendations in the United States?

   A. The human papillomavirus (HPV) immunization is recommended for females ages 6–12 years.
   B. Adolescents should receive initial immunoprophylaxis against *Neisseria meningitidis* between ages 6 and 12 years.

C. The meningococcal conjugate polysaccharide vaccine (MCV4) is preferable to the meningococcal polysaccharide vaccine (MPSV4) unless there are contraindications.
D. Immunoprophylaxis against HPV is recommended to reduce the incidence of genital warts.

Clinical Case 11

Ms. Cooper is a 27-year-old female with major depressive disorder and a remote suicide attempt. Her illness is in remission with sertraline, and she presents for routine medication management. She is accompanied today by her children, ages 13 months and 3 years. She states that she fears her children may someday suffer from the same illness that almost took her life.

1. In addressing Ms. Cooper's concerns about her children's well-being, which of the following should you advise her is the leading cause of death for children and adolescents?

   A. Suicide.
   B. Homicide.
   C. Overdose.
   D. Accidental injury.

2. If Ms. Cooper places her children in safety seats, that would reduce risk of fatality in a motor vehicle accident by what percent?

   A. 20%.
   B. 40%.
   C. 60%.
   D. 80%.

3. What is the leading cause of mortality in infants?

   A. Suffocation.
   B. Sudden infant death syndrome.
   C. Gun violence.
   D. Heat stroke associated with parked cars.

SECTION VIII

Pain Medicine in the Psychiatric Patient Population

Section Editor:
Robert M. McCarron, D.O., DFAPA

Kristian Delgado, M.D.

With

Naileshni Singh, M.D.

Amir Ramezani, Ph.D.

Matthew Reed, M.D., M.S.P.H.

CHAPTER 27

Pain Medicine

Clinical Case 1

Ms. Castro is a 42-year-old woman with axial back pain. She has been taking opioids for the past 5 years. While she was returning home from a trip to Italy, she lost her medications. She reports that shortly thereafter, she began to experience muscle aches, abdominal cramping, diarrhea, and rhinorrhea.

1. Which of the following best describes the patient's current state?

    A. Physical dependence.
    B. Tolerance.
    C. Addiction.
    D. Abuse.

2. Further investigation reveals that this is not the first time that Ms. Castro has called in for lost medications. There is concern that the patient is obtaining opioids from other sources. What would be the most appropriate next step?

    A. Write a prescription for the opioids.
    B. Deny the patient further opioid therapy.
    C. Review the Prescription Drug Monitoring Program (PDMP) database.
    D. Discharge the patient from your practice.

3. At the end of the week, the patient returns to your clinic for evaluation. She is sweaty, has dilated pupils and slightly elevated blood

pressure, and appears intoxicated. What is the most appropriate next step?

A. Perform an electrocardiogram.
B. Order a computed tomographic (CT) scan of the head.
C. Check a urine drug screen.
D. Check cardiac enzymes.
E. Order a pulmonary angiogram.

Clinical Case 2

Ms. Wilson is a 42-year-old obese black woman with fibromyalgia who presents to your clinic for an initial evaluation. She has a past medical history of hypertension, type 2 diabetes, and hypercholesterolemia.

1. Which of the following of Ms. Wilson's statements may be assessed using the AMPS approach to psychiatric illness?

   A. "When I sleep, my husband can hear me snore from the next room."
   B. "I was an alcoholic for 12 years."
   C. "On a scale from 1 to 10, I rate my pain 5 most days of the week."
   D. "Most nights I only sleep 4 hours because I wake up gasping for air."
   E. "I frequently run out of oxycodone before it is time for my refill."

2. Ms. Wilson has been undergoing several months of physical therapy, stretching, and meditation exercises, which had provided significant relief from her shoulder pain until recently. Currently, her pain, which she rates 5 of 10 on the visual analog scale (VAS), is unrelieved with these actions. She has not taken any type of medications. What would be your next step according to the World Health Organization's three-step analgesic ladder?

   A. Try treatment with a short-acting opioid and a nonsteroidal anti-inflammatory drug (NSAID).
   B. Try treatment with a long-acting opioid.
   C. Try treatment with an NSAID for 1 week and then add a short-acting opioid.
   D. Recommend further lifestyle modification.
   E. Try treatment with a topical anesthetic.

3. At Ms. Wilson's next clinic visit, she reports no improvement in symptoms after a trial with a topical anesthetic. Prior to considering an

additional medication, which of the following needs to be performed before you make your decision?

A. Urine drug screen.
B. 2- to 4-week minimal duration trials of medications.
C. PDMP database search.
D. Interventional pain procedures if indicated.
E. Answers B and D.
F. All of the above.

4. Ms. Wilson has a body mass index (BMI) greater than 35 and hypertension. The presence of which additional factor would put the patient at high risk for obstructive sleep apnea?

A. Neck circumference of 36 cm.
B. Age less than 50 years.
C. Quiet snoring.
D. Nighttime tiredness.

Clinical Case 3

Mr. Bateman is a 54-year-old HIV-positive man who has been undergoing antiretroviral therapy for the past 20 years. He presents to your clinic as a new consultation and complains about "pins and needles" pain in both hands and rhinorrhea. His pain medication has been titrated up to 400 mg/day of morphine equivalents over the past 4 years. He is a recovering alcoholic and last used methamphetamine 5 days ago.

1. What would be the most appropriate next step before deciding how to proceed with treatment?

A. Check a CD4 count.
B. Check the PDMP database.
C. Check liver function tests.
D. Check a urine drug screen.
E. Answers B and D.

2. The "pins and needles" pain that the patient is experiencing is best described as which of the following?

A. Somatic pain.
B. Referred somatic pain.
C. Visceral pain.

D. Nociceptive pain.
E. Neuropathic pain.

3. In addition to the 400 mg/day of morphine equivalents, the patient also takes gabapentin 900 mg/day, acetaminophen 2 g/day, and diazepam 5 mg hs for sleep. With the patient's current medication regimen, which of the following is he most at risk for?

    A. Tolerance.
    B. Hyperalgesia.
    C. Loss of bone mineral density.
    D. Accidental death.
    E. All of the above.

Clinical Case 4

Ms. Aterman is a 32-year-old woman with obstructive sleep apnea, hypertension, uncontrolled type 2 diabetes, and fibromyalgia. The patient reports to you that she has good pain relief and increased daily activity while on opioids. She drinks one glass of wine nightly and smokes one cigarette daily. She does not use her continuous positive airway pressure (CPAP) machine regularly.

1. Which of the following is important for the assessment of opioid management in this patient?

    A. Tobacco and alcohol use.
    B. Poor CPAP compliance.
    C. Adequate pain relief and increased daily activity.
    D. Uncontrolled type 2 diabetes.

2. While using the AMPS tool to assess for comorbid psychiatric illness, you discover that Ms. Aterman was an avid painter but does not enjoy painting anymore. She also reports poor sleep and loss of energy. The patient exhibits symptoms of which of the following that can make her pain worse?

    A. Anxiety.
    B. Depression.
    C. Mania.
    D. Psychosis.
    E. Substance misuse.

3. Ms. Aterman returns for a follow-up visit in your clinic 6 months after you last saw her. She did not show up for her two previously scheduled visits and did not cancel her appointments. When you query the PDMP database, you discover that she has several opioid prescriptions from other providers as well as from the emergency department, and has contacted your office for early opioid refills several times over the past few months. Which of the following is a possible explanation for her behavior?

   A. Opioid abuse.
   B. Diversion.
   C. Lost medication.
   D. Answers A and B.
   E. All of the above.

4. Which of the following is most the appropriate monitoring for high-risk patients?

   A. Urine drug screen once a year.
   B. Urine drug screens monthly.
   C. Urine drug screens every 3–6 months.
   D. PDMP database review for new prescriptions only.
   E. PDMP database review three times a year.

Clinical Case 5

Ms. Davis is a 34-year-old woman with no significant past medical history who sustained a whiplash injury from a motor vehicle collision last year, which causes waxing and waning neck pain. Since the accident she experiences repeated vivid memories of the accident, sleeps poorly, and avoids using the same route where the accident occurred. Ms. Davis feels detached and frequently avoids social situations.

1. Which of the following can be a potential amplifier of the patient's pain?

   A. Poor blood glucose control.
   B. Poor compliance with medical care.
   C. Untreated anxiety.
   D. Occasional alcohol use.

2. Ms. Davis has been taking an antidepressant and an NSAID for several months with no appreciable improvement in symptoms. You are considering a trial of a short-acting opioid for the patient. Which of the following needs to be done prior to initiating this therapy?

   A. No further actions.
   B. Trial a different NSAID.
   C. Start a long-acting opioid.
   D. Longer trial of current medications.

3. Ms. Davis has been taking a short-acting opioid for approximately 1 year. She initially received pain relief on a low dose of morphine but has been requiring higher doses to obtain the same therapeutic benefit. What is most likely happening?

   A. Dependence.
   B. Addiction.
   C. Tolerance.
   D. Abuse.
   E. Diversion.

4. Ms. Davis has been using an increased dose of sustained-release morphine product for baseline pain control for about 14 months. She also uses an immediate-release morphine formulation for breakthrough pain every 6 hours. The addition of a benzodiazepine for muscle spasms would put the patient at risk for which of the following?

   A. Hyperalgesia.
   B. Tolerance.
   C. Loss of bone mineral density.
   D. Accidental death.
   E. Suppression of sex steroids.

Clinical Case 6

Ms. Bradford is a morbidly obese 42-year-old woman who presents to your clinic with headaches, general body aches, weight gain, fatigue, and depression.

1. Which of the following tests would be most beneficial in determining the patient's pathology?

   A. Blood glucose.
   B. Thyroid-stimulating hormone test.

C. Head and neck CT scan.
D. Complete blood count.
E. Liver function tests.

2. Ms. Bradford snores loudly at night and frequently wakes up her housemate. She weighs 260 lbs, is 5 feet 4 inches tall, and has a neck circumference of 34 inches. There have been no witnessed apneic episodes when she falls asleep on the couch, and the patient is frequently tired in the daytime. Which of the above findings demonstrate(s) that the patient needs additional studies by a sleep specialist?

   A. Loud snoring.
   B. Calculated BMI.
   C. Daytime somnolence.
   D. Female sex.
   E. Answers A, B, and C.

3. When you perform a physical examination of Ms. Bradford, you find multiple tight ropelike muscle bands over the periscapular and trapezius muscles. Palpation of these bands causes her to feel pain in other locations. Which intervention would be most appropriate for this patient?

   A. Radiofrequency ablation of the medial branch nerves.
   B. Epidural steroid injections.
   C. Facet steroid injections.
   D. Trigger point injections.

Clinical Case 7

Mr. Sidel is a 53-year-old man with hypertension, grade II obesity (BMI> 35), and chronic paranoid schizophrenia being treated with olanzapine monotherapy, who presents to the clinic for psychiatric follow-up. He is stable from a psychiatric standpoint but complains of persistent lateral leg and foot pain from known lumbar radiculopathy. He tried gabapentin but discontinued it due to sedative side effects. He continues to feel fatigued during the day despite sleeping 8–10 hours per night, but he is most concerned about his pain. He has declined epidural steroid injections and is discussing a trial of short-acting opioids with his primary care physician.

1. Which potentially serious medical condition should be ruled out prior to starting an opiate medication?

A. Coronary artery disease.
B. Diabetes.
C. Obstructive sleep apnea.
D. Hyperlipidemia.

2. Which of the following acronyms represents a screening tool for the medical condition referred to in the previous question?

A. A-SCAR.
B. STOP-BANG.
C. VITAMIN D.
D. CREATE.

3. Following a thorough sleep and sleep apnea assessment, what would you recommend to Mr. Sidel's primary care provider?

A. A trial of an opiate medication.
B. Retrial of gabapentin at a lower dose.
C. Referral for a sleep study.
D. A trial of tramadol.

Clinical Case 8

Mr. Vincent is an 82-year-old Russian-speaking man with coronary artery disease who is seen regularly in the internal medicine clinic for angina. You note that Mr. Vincent is a high resource utilizer and is seen almost monthly in the emergency department for chest pain. He is frequently admitted to the cardiac care unit for monitoring. His medical assessments for acute ischemia, pulmonary embolism, or any other cardiac etiology are negative. On interview, the patient focuses on his blood pressure control and notes that he measures his blood pressure at least four times daily. He describes constant concern that he will have a heart attack and has been limiting his activities to prevent provoking his chest pain.

1. Which area of psychiatric pathology evaluated using the AMPS psychiatric assessment is likely contributing to Mr. Vincent's chest pain?

A. Anxiety.
B. Mood.
C. Psychosis.
D. Substance abuse.

2. Which of the following nonpharmacological therapies for the treatment of pain would be most appropriate for this patient?

   A. Physical therapy.
   B. Acupuncture.
   C. Meditation.
   D. Cognitive-behavioral therapy.

3. How can anxiety maintain pain and limit the effectiveness of pain interventions?

   A. By intensifying the sympathetic response.
   B. By adversely affecting sleep.
   C. By causing the patient to feign symptoms.
   D. By hurting the doctor-patient relationship.
   E. Answers A and B.

Clinical Case 9

Ms. Juglar is a 43-year-old woman who is overweight (BMI = 28) and who has an unspecified mood disorder. She presents to your clinic for psychiatric follow-up. Over the last few months, she has consistently described three "knots" in her back that are exquisitely tender to palpation, with radiating sharp pain to her gluteal area. The pain is making it difficult for her to work the long hours her desk job requires. She is concerned that she may have to find a new job. She refuses to see her primary care physician because "the only thing he will suggest is that I see a physical therapist."

1. Which of the following is the most likely diagnosis?

   A. Disc herniation with radicular pain.
   B. Facet arthropathy.
   C. Fibromyalgia.
   D. Myofascial pain syndrome.

2. Besides physical therapy, massage, and ultrasound, which of the following interventional modalities is commonly used to treat myofascial pain syndrome?

   A. Radiofrequency ablation.
   B. Trigger point injection.
   C. Epidural steroid injection.
   D. Sympathetic block.

3. Many patients have myofascial tenderness to palpation, which is not classified as a trigger point. Which of the following is required for the diagnosis of a trigger point?

   A. Hyperirritable spot with referred symptoms.
   B. Multiple points of tenderness throughout the body.
   C. Radicular spine pain.
   D. Motor or autonomic dysfunction.

Clinical Case 10

Ms. Palmer, a 67-year-old woman with poorly controlled type 2 diabetes, hypertension, obesity (grade II), and recently diagnosed major depressive disorder, is presenting for her initial evaluation in the psychiatry clinic. She was referred by her primary care physician who started the patient on mirtazapine 30 mg qhs last month. In the course of your evaluation, you discover that her depressive symptoms have been exacerbated by a progressive loss of function caused by bilateral lower extremity pain. She describes the pain as burning with some numbness and tingling in a stocking distribution. She has been taking ibuprofen and acetaminophen with minimal benefit. Her primary care physician has not yet trialed a pain medication.

1. What is the most likely cause of Ms. Palmer's lower extremity pain?

   A. Spondylolisthesis.
   B. Degenerative disc disease.
   C. Diabetic peripheral neuropathy.
   D. Fibromyalgia.

2. Which of the following medications would be a first-line recommendation for Ms. Palmer's pain condition and depressive disorder?

   A. Duloxetine.
   B. Amitriptyline.
   C. Gabapentin.
   D. Sertraline.

3. How might treatment with mirtazapine worsen her medical conditions?

   A. By worsening her depression.
   B. By increasing sensitivity to neuropathic pain.
   C. By increasing appetite.
   D. By impairing sleep.

Clinical Case 11

Mr. Whitcomb is a 54-year-old man with bipolar I disorder, peptic ulcer disease (well controlled with a proton pump inhibitor), and chronic axial lower back pain who presents to your clinic for psychiatric follow-up. Mr. Whitcomb has not experienced a manic episode in more than 2 years; his mood is currently stable with lithium maintenance therapy. Today, he complains of chronic axial lower back pain that is not radiating. The pain has worsened over the past 4 months. He has not seen his primary care provider in over a year and is hesitant to see his provider because "they can't do anything for lower back pain anyway." The pain is most noticeable when he extends and/or rotates his back. He denies any lower extremity numbness, paresthesia, or weakness.

1. Based on the patient's history, which of the following is the most likely diagnosis?

   A. Disc herniation.
   B. Lumbar facet arthropathy.
   C. Spinal stenosis.
   D. Diabetic neuropathy.

2. Which analgesic class is typically recommended first for the treatment of this patient's pain?

   A. NSAID.
   B. Opiate.
   C. Anticonvulsant.
   D. SNRI.

3. Mr. Whitcomb has peptic ulcer disease and is unable to take NSAIDs. In this situation, which of the following interventional procedures is commonly used to treat his kind of back pain?

   A. Transcutaneous electrical nerve stimulation (TENS).
   B. Epidural steroid injection.
   C. Trigger point injection.
   D. Radiofrequency ablation.

Clinical Case 12

Ms. Schulte is a 52-year-old woman with type 2 diabetes (with peripheral neuropathy), hypertension, grade III obesity (BMI≥40), bilateral osteoarthritis of the knees, and recurrent major depressive disorder who was referred by her primary care physician to the psychiatry clinic for evaluation of worsening depression. The patient is tearful about her inability to get out of the house and find work. She cites pain with ambulation and fatigue as the reasons for her immobility. Her pain is localized in her knees. She denies significant burning, numbness, or tingling in her feet. She feels "constantly exhausted" and naps throughout the day. Her medications include gabapentin 600 mg tid, OxyContin (controlled-release oxycodone) 15 mg q12h, oxycodone 5–10 mg q6h, insulin glargine 60 units qhs, insulin aspart 10 units tid with meals, metoprolol 25 mg bid, hydrochlorothiazide 25 mg qam, and paroxetine 20 mg qam.

1. Which of the patient's medications represents the greatest risk for respiratory depression?

   A. Gabapentin.
   B. Oxycodone.
   C. Paroxetine.
   D. Insulin glargine.

2. The knee pain Ms. Schulte experiences with ambulation is most consistent with bilateral osteoarthritis. Which of the following nonpharmacological therapies should be part of her comprehensive pain treatment program?

   A. Weight loss guidance.
   B. TENS.
   C. Yoga.
   D. Acupuncture.

3. Which of the following choices contains the two most likely reasons for Ms. Schulte's fatigue?

   A. Ruminating thoughts at night and sedentary lifestyle.
   B. Obstructive sleep apnea and worsened pain at night.
   C. Sedentary lifestyle and multiple sedating medications.
   D. Obstructive sleep apnea and multiple sedating medications.
   E. Worsened pain at night and ruminating thoughts at night.

PART 2

ANSWER GUIDE

CHAPTER 1

Medical Comorbidities and Behavioral Health

Clinical Case 1

1. **The correct response is option C: He is more likely to get pneumonia and influenza.**

   Patients with severe mental illness are three to four times more likely to die from chronic obstructive pulmonary disease (COPD). Respiratory symptoms are not common delusions in people with bipolar disorder. Persons with this disorder are more likely to develop potentially life-threatening respiratory infections such as pneumonia and influenza. It is possible that mania could lead to hyperventilation, but this is not a common cause of a cough or shortness of breath. **(p. 5)**

2. **The correct response is option C: They consume more than one-third of all tobacco products.**

   People with severe mental illness are more likely to get pneumonia and influenza, in part because they are less likely to utilize or have access to preventive health services, including pulmonary-related vaccinations. The influenza vaccine is unlikely to cause significant respiratory problems. Estimates are that 50%–80% of patients with severe mental illness smoke tobacco. A study has shown that patients with severe mental illness smoke more than one-third of available tobacco products. Respiratory infections occur more frequently in the fall and winter and may be associated with spending time indoors and in low-humidity environments. **(pp. 5, 8)**

3. **The correct response is option A: He was at higher risk of developing metabolic syndrome and related vascular disease.**

   People with severe mental illness have a much higher risk of developing metabolic syndrome. They are less likely to receive invasive cardiovascular procedures such as coronary artery bypass grafting or angioplasty and stenting. Additionally, they are less likely to receive therapies proven to decrease major coronary events such as angiotensin-converting enzyme inhibitors. **(pp. 5, 8)**

4. **The correct response is option B: Antipsychotics vary greatly with regard to metabolic risk.**

   Antipsychotics have different effects on weight and metabolic outcomes, and the options should be carefully considered when you are deciding which agent to use. Even though a patient may be stabilized when taking a specific medication, it is reasonable to consider gradually switching to a medication with lower risk of metabolic side effects. A dose-response relationship exists between olanzapine and metabolic outcomes. Sodium valproate may cause significant weight gain. **(pp. 6–7)**

Clinical Case 2

1. **The correct response is option A: Less than 25%.**

   There is good evidence that many atypical antipsychotics worsen cardiovascular and metabolic conditions. The Clinical Antipsychotic Trials of Intervention Effectiveness (CATIE) study showed that 88% of patients taking antipsychotics do not receive the standard of care for hypertension management. **(p. 6)**

2. **The correct response is option B: She is more likely to have died from natural causes than from suicide or injury.**

   Patients with severe mental illness are likely to die 13–30 years earlier than the general population of the United States. Approximately 60% of the excess mortality in patients with schizophrenia can be attributed to cardiovascular disease, diabetes, respiratory disease, and other infections. This increased risk of mortality is related in part to a lack of primary and preventive medical care. **(pp. 3, 5)**

3. **The correct response is option A: Her Framingham Cardiovascular Risk Score was likely similar to that of a woman 10–15 years older in the general population.**

   In a Spanish cohort study it was found that the cardiovascular risk (using the Framingham Cardiovascular Risk Score) of patients with severe mental illness was similar to that of people in the general population who were 10–15 years older. People with severe mental illness are five and seven times more likely to die from diabetes and hepatitis C, respectively. **(p. 5)**

Clinical Case 3

1. **The correct response is option E: Answers A, B, and C.**

   Monitoring waist circumference after a patient begins taking risperidone should be a top priority and may predict severe risk for vascular disease. Thyroid dysfunction can exacerbate mood disturbances and lithium can lead to thyroid dysfunction, so it is important to check a patient's thyroid-stimulating hormone serum level. It is reasonable to expect mental health providers to check hemoglobin A_{1c} because psychiatric patients are disproportionately affected by diabetes. These patients should also be screened and referred for hepatitis C, which disproportionately affects psychiatric patients and can worsen mood disorders. However, making hepatitis C treatment decisions is not normally within the standard of care for most psychiatrists. **(pp. 5, 8)**

2. **The correct response is option C: A 30-year-old woman with bipolar I disorder and hypertension.**

   Patient A would be categorized in Quadrant I for having mild to moderate physical and mental health problems (Figure 1–1). Patient B would be in Quadrant III for having mild to moderate mental and moderate to severe physical health problems. Both Patients A and B are mainly served by the primary health care system. Patient C would be in Quadrant II for having mild to moderate physical and moderate to severe mental health problems and would benefit most from preventive medicine to reduce progression. Although Patient D is the most mentally and physically ill overall (Quadrant IV), Patient C is more likely to benefit from intervention. **(p. 10)**

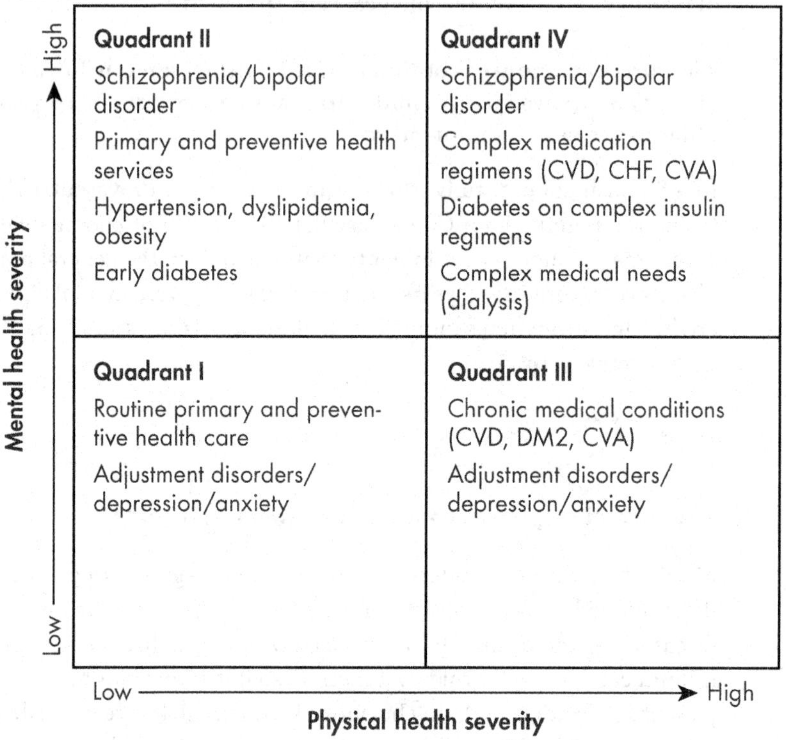

FIGURE 1–1. The Four-Quadrant Clinical Integration Model.

Note. CHF=congestive heart failure; CVA = cerebrovascular accident; CVD = cardiovascular disease; DM2=diabetes mellitus type 2.

Source. Adapted from Center for Integrated Health Solutions: *Four Quadrant Model.* Washington, DC, National Council for Community Behavioral Healthcare. Available at: http://www.integration.samhsa.gov/resource/four-quadrant-model. Accessed July 7, 2014; Mauer J: *Behavioral Health/Primary Care Integration: The Four Quadrant Model and Evidence-Based Practices.* Rockville, MD, National Council for Community Behavioral Healthcare, February 2006; Parks J, Pollack D, Bartels S, et al.: *Integrating Behavioral Health and Primary Care Services: Opportunities and Challenges for State Mental Health Authorities.* Alexandria, VA, National Association of State Mental Health Program Directors (NASMHPD) Medical Directors Council, 2005.

3. **The correct response is option D: All of the above.**

Collaborative care improves health outcomes by addressing the physical health of those with severe mental illness. Three key components of collaborative care models are 1) locating primary care services in or near mental health organizations, 2) linking patients to services, and 3) promoting health or wellness activities. **(p. 11)**

4. **The correct response is option E: Answers A and C.**

   The Affordable Care Act permits health homes to be established in behavioral health settings for patients with severe mental illness. These health homes are not funded to provide direct primary care but should provide core services to improve health outcomes. These services include care management and coordination, health promotion, transitional care between facilities, individual and family support, and community and social support services. **(pp. 11–12)**

CHAPTER 2

Fundamentals of Preventive Care

Clinical Case 1

1. **The correct response is option C: Counsel her on smoking cessation.**

   Preventive care comprises screening, counseling on lifestyle changes, immunizations, and preventive medications. Mrs. Johnson is already taking appropriate cardioprotective pharmacological therapy. Smoking increases her risk for another myocardial infarction or cerebrovascular accident. Smoking cessation would greatly decrease this risk and is the most important *reversible* cardiovascular risk factor. There is no evidence that doses of atorvastatin higher than 80 mg/day have increased benefits. Increasing aspirin to 325 mg could increase risk of bleeding with no added benefit. There are no indications at this time to change her antidepressive regimen. **(p. 15)**

2. **The correct response is option C: Tertiary prevention.**

   The goal of tertiary prevention is to mitigate further consequences of disease. This type of prevention makes up the majority of "chronic disease management." Primary prevention focuses on preventing new disease from occurring by removing causes. Secondary prevention involves detecting diseases in early stages before the patient has any symptoms. Because Mrs. Johnson already has coronary artery disease, she is at higher risk for future events. β-Blockers, angiotensin-converting enzyme inhibitors, lipid-lowering agents, and aspirin have all been proven to reduce further cardiovascular events after a myocardial infarction. **(p. 16)**

3. **The correct response is option B: Secondary prevention.**

   Secondary prevention involves detecting diseases in early stages before the patient has any symptoms. Detection at this stage has a major role in preventing disease progression. Primary prevention focuses on preventing new disease from occurring by removing causes. Diagnostic testing refers to testing for a disease in someone who is already manifesting symptoms of disease. **(p. 16)**

Clinical Case 2

1. **The correct response is option C: You should look for updated screening guidelines from a source such as National Guideline Clearinghouse (www.guideline.gov).**

   To find preventive practice recommendations, a practicing provider should perform a simple Web or PubMed search for the condition in question. For example, in regard to pap smears, the American Cancer Society, U.S. Preventive Services Task Force (USPSTF), and American College of Obstetricians and Gynecologists currently recommend cervical cancer screening with pap smears every 3 years or screening with a pap smear and human papillomavirus testing every 5 years for asymptomatic average-risk women ages 30–65 years. These guidelines tend to change often. The National Guideline Clearinghouse provides a searchable database at www.guideline.gov for updated evidence-based guidelines. **(pp. 17–18)**

2. **The correct response is option A: This service should be offered only to selected patients because the net benefit is likely to be small.**

   For grade C evidence, the USPSTF recommends selectively offering a service based on professional judgment and patient preferences because the net benefit is likely to be small (Table 2–1). **(p. 19)**

3. **The correct response is option E: There is insufficient evidence to offer or discourage this service.**

   For grade I evidence, the USPSTF concludes that there is insufficient evidence to assess the benefits and harms of the service. Patients should understand that there is uncertainty if this service is performed (see Table 2–1). **(p. 19)**

TABLE 2–1. U.S. Preventive Services Task Force (USPSTF) grading system

Grade	Definition	Suggestions for practice
A	The USPSTF recommends the service. There is high certainty that the net benefit is substantial.	Offer or provide this service.
B	The USPSTF recommends the service. There is high certainty that the net benefit is moderate or there is moderate certainty that the net benefit is moderate to substantial.	Offer or provide this service.
C	The USPSTF recommends selectively offering or providing this service to individual patients based on professional judgment and patient preferences. There is at least moderate certainty that the net benefit is small.	Offer or provide this service for selected patients depending on individual circumstances.
D	The USPSTF recommends against the service. There is moderate or high certainty that the service has no net benefit or that the harms outweigh the benefits.	Discourage the use of this service.
I Statement	The USPSTF concludes that the current evidence is insufficient to assess the balance of benefits and harms of the service. Evidence is lacking, of poor quality, or conflicting, and the balance of benefits and harms cannot be determined.	Read the clinical considerations section of the USPSTF recommendation statement. If the service is offered, patients should understand the uncertainty about the balance of benefits and harms.

Source. U.S. Preventive Services Task Force Grade Definitions. July 2012. Available at: https://www.uspreventiveservicestaskforce.org/Page/Name/grade-definitions.

4. **The correct response is option C: This service should be offered, and the net benefit is likely to be at least moderate.**

For grade B evidence, the USPSTF recommends offering the service (see Table 2–1). There is either high certainty that the benefit is moderate or moderate certainty that the benefit is moderate to substantial. **(p. 19)**

Clinical Case 3

1. **The correct response is option C: Ordering a hemoglobin A_{1c} test.**

   Because Mr. Carson has a history of obesity, hypertension, extensive smoking, and chronic exposure to olanzapine, he is at increased risk for developing metabolic syndrome and diabetes mellitus. Ordering a hemoglobin A_{1c} test is a secondary prevention measure, which would detect diabetes or prediabetes before the patient becomes symptomatic. Taking antihypertensive medication to prevent myocardial infarction or stroke and having yearly influenza vaccines are two examples of primary prevention. Primary prevention focuses on preventing new disease from occurring by removing causes. Using topiramate for weight loss is not common practice; the first step to weight loss is a combination of diet and exercise. Starting metformin would be an example of tertiary prevention, with goals of preventing complications from diabetes such as renal failure, neuropathy, and retinopathy. **(p. 16)**

2. **The correct response is option B: Secondary prevention.**

   The goal of secondary prevention is to detect diseases in early stages while individuals are asymptomatic and when treatment can prevent disease progression. Helping Mr. Carson with weight loss can help prevent worsening metabolic syndrome, diabetes, and increased risk for cardiovascular events. **(p. 16)**

3. **The correct response is option B: Screening must be able to identify a disease that becomes clinically significant if left untreated.**

   For a screening program to be effective, it must meet certain minimum standards, as listed in Table 2–2. **(p. 17)**

TABLE 2–2. Essential criteria for an effective screening program

The screening test must identify a disease that becomes clinically significant if left untreated.
The screening test must be able to detect the disease in a preclinical stage.
The disease in question must be treatable, so that finding it and treating it early will lead to reduced morbidity or mortality.

TABLE 2–2.	**Essential criteria for an effective screening program *(continued)***

The test must have acceptable sensitivity and specificity in order to avoid high false-positive rates (to avoid unnecessary testing) and false-negative test results (to be effective at finding early disease).

The ideal screening test is reasonably priced, so it can be applied widely, and poses minimal harm or discomfort to the patient.

Clinical Case 4

1. **The correct response is option E: All of the above.**

   Mr. Lee has not yet manifested symptoms of chronic medical disease. However, he is at high risk of developing metabolic syndrome (characterized by hyperlipidemia, obesity, increased waist circumference, hypertension, and glucose intolerance) and cardiovascular events given his smoking history, serious mental illness, and quetiapine use. A lipid panel, hemoglobin A_{1c} test, and measure of waist circumference are all screening measures for metabolic syndrome. Smoking significantly increases cardiovascular risks. The USPSTF recommends HIV screening for adults ages 15–65 years at least one time and more frequently for persons with increased risk. **(p. 16)**

2. **The correct response is option D: Counsel him on smoking cessation.**

   HIV screening and measuring cholesterol and A_{1c} levels are examples of secondary prevention because they focus on preventing disease progression in asymptomatic individuals. Smoking cessation counseling is a primary prevention activity because it focuses on preventing a new disease, such as lung cancer, from occurring by removing its cause. **(p. 16)**

3. **The correct response is option A: Implement all the preventive care interventions at one visit.**

   Mr. Lee is a relatively healthy young patient with stable psychiatric symptoms and a number of cardiovascular risk factors given his smoking history and quetiapine therapy. Because he comes to the clinic infrequently, he may miss opportunities for preventive care. An annual visit that covers all screening appropriate for his age and risk factors would likely be longer than his previous visits, but it is the best way to offer comprehensive care for this individual. If Mr. Lee were to come to the clinic regularly, it would be reasonable to systematically perform a small amount of preventive care throughout several shorter visits. **(pp. 18–20)**

CHAPTER 3

Cultural Considerations in Psychiatry

Clinical Case 1

1. **The correct response is option B: She will be more likely to accept assessment and recommendations and to follow up with preventive medical care.**

   There is no evidence that addressing an individual's culture worsens hypertension. Ignoring cultural perspectives may result in worse outcomes in areas such as preventive screening and delayed immunizations and eventually lead to increased mortality. Cultural humility facilitates stronger therapeutic relationships and better outcomes. **(p. 24)**

2. **The correct response is option A: Ask the patient what she thinks is happening.**

   An open-ended approach, as described in option A, allows the patient the opportunity to share her experience of the illness, which may give the clinician information about the patient's cultural conceptualization of distress and psychosocial stressors. *Ataque de nervios* is a syndrome of a wide range of symptoms of distress commonly associated with individuals of Latino descent. Although it is a possible explanation for her symptoms, the patient will be best served through exploring possibilities and establishing rapport. Because hypertension is common and often asymptomatic early in its course, there is no need to question her about not having had prior treatment. Providing a benzodiazepine may provide temporary relief of anxiety, but is unlikely to treat the underlying issue. **(pp. 25, 27)**

3. **The correct response is option A: Work together with the *curandero* to form a treatment plan.**

   It is important to collaborate with a trusted cultural broker in order to establish relationships and help navigate complex scenarios. Using a family member or untrained translator for a medical encounter will more likely lead to misunderstanding, poor follow-up, or medical errors. Scare tactics have limited utility in encouraging long-term adherence. **(p. 25)**

Clinical Case 2

1. **The correct response is option A: Compared with nonminorities, they are more likely to have worse outcomes, including increased mortality.**

   Minorities have less access to and receive a lower quality of physical and mental health care, which results in worse outcomes including increased mortality. Ethnic minority populations are rapidly growing in the United States. A multicultural approach is a reciprocal learning experience with emphasis on understanding the patient's perspective so that a relationship develops and the provider may better meet the patient's needs. **(pp. 23–24)**

2. **The correct response is option D: All of the above.**

   Options A, B, and C are all included in the CREATE cultural competence mnemonic (Table 3–1). **(p. 25)**

Clinical Case 3

1. **The correct response is option D: Answers A and C.**

   Cultural conceptualization of distress describes the construct that shapes a person's understanding and experience of his or her problems and symptoms. Understanding the patient's beliefs regarding his or

TABLE 3–1. CREATE cultural competence

Collaborate with a cultural broker when encountering complex, culturally influenced medical situations.
Reflect on your own cultural beliefs and how they may affect the treatment plan.
Empathize with the patient's cultural belief system, even if you do not fully understand or agree with a particular belief or related behavior.
Ancillary staff should be trained about CREATE, as they are often the first and last to interact with patients at each medical encounter.
Timing of specific culturally related stressors to illness may help the provider conceptualize and diagnose the clinical problem more accurately.
Educate yourself about commonly encountered cultures (e.g., religions and ethnicities).

her disease is important for engaging the patient with a treatment plan. Race and ethnicity, religion and spirituality, gender and sexual orientation, and socioeconomic status are all important cultural factors to address while making a treatment plan. **(pp. 24–26)**

2. **The correct response is option E: Answers A, B, and C.**

   DSM-5 provides an overall cultural assessment, the Cultural Formulation Interview (CFI), that can help in identifying the cultural factors that impact a person's health. Table 3–2 is a shortened version of the CFI that provides high-yield questions for practical use in clinical settings. The CFI encompasses questions that help identify 1) cultural definition of the problem; 2) cultural perception of cause, context, and support; 3) role of cultural identity; and 4) cultural factors affecting self-coping and past help seeking. **(pp. 26–27)**

3. **The correct response is option C: Consult with a *houngan* in your community to work together to treat her depression.**

   The CREATE cultural competence model (see Table 3–1) encourages clinicians to collaborate with cultural brokers to help navigate through complex and culturally influenced medical situations. By consulting with such an authority, the clinician shows that he or she considers the patient's culture to be important. This merging of the patient's belief system with the physician's biochemical and therapeutic models of illness may increase the likelihood that the patient will understand and adhere to treatment. **(p. 25)**

TABLE 3–2. Cultural Formulation Interview

Cultural Definition of the Problem

1. What troubles you most about your problem?

Cultural Perceptions of Cause, Context, and Support

2. Why do you think this is happening to you? What do you think are the causes of your [PROBLEM]?
3. Are there any kinds of supports that make your [PROBLEM] better, such as from family, friends, or others?
4. Are there any kinds of stresses that make your [PROBLEM] worse, such as difficulties with money, or family problems?

Role of Cultural Identity

Sometimes, aspects of people's background or identity can make the [PROBLEM] better or worse. By *background* or *identity,* I mean, for example, the communities you belong to, the languages you speak, where you or your family are from, your race or ethnic background, your gender or sexual orientation, and your faith or religion.

5. For you, what are the most important aspects of your background or identity?

Cultural Factors Affecting Self-Coping and Past Help Seeking

6. Sometimes people have various ways of dealing with problems like [PROBLEM]. What have you done on your own to cope with your [PROBLEM]?
7. Has anything prevented you from getting the help you need?
8. What kinds of help would be most useful to you at this time for your [PROBLEM]?

Source. Adapted from American Psychiatric Association: *Diagnostic and Statistical Manual of Mental Disorders,* 5th Edition. Arlington, VA, American Psychiatric Association, 2013, pp. 750–754.

CHAPTER 4

Preventive Medicine and Psychiatric Training Considerations

Clinical Case 1

1. **The correct response is option E: All of the above.**

   Research has demonstrated that a variety of approaches can help to improve medical outcomes in the mental health sector. In some models, being assigned to a nurse manager increases the chance that a patient will have a primary care physician (PCP) and receive recommended preventive services. Other studies have shown that a PCP colocated into a mental health clinic results in increased primary care visits and improved target goal attainment for blood pressure, lipids, and body mass index. Multiple studies have shown that collaborative care improves health in patients with comorbid diabetes and depression in terms of increased adherence, remission rates, quality of life, functional status, and patient satisfaction in primary care settings. **(p. 34)**

2. **The correct response is option C: 8 years earlier.**

   Patients with mental disorders die an average of 8.2 years earlier than the rest of the population. Excess mortality is due to socioeconomic factors, poor access to effective primary care and preventive health care, and chronic health conditions. Patients with schizophrenia die

20–30 years earlier than the general population, and those with bipolar disorder have a twofold higher mortality rate. Earlier mortality is largely attributable to natural causes, primarily cardiovascular disease. **(p. 32)**

3. **The correct response is option D: All of the above.**

   Patients with depression are at higher risk for myocardial infarction as well as general medical illness. Earlier detection and prevention of medical illness in patients with psychiatric disorders has been shown to decrease mortality. **(p. 32)**

Clinical Case 2

1. **The correct response is option B: A nurse manager who works with a psychiatrist and PCP in a collaborative team.**

   Multiple studies have shown that collaborative care groups lead to improved health outcomes for patients with comorbid diabetes and depression. Studies have shown that patients who have been assigned a nurse care manager were more likely to have a PCP and to receive a higher percentage of recommended preventive and cardiometabolic interventions. Nurse care managers provide health education, motivational interviewing, coaching on how to interact effectively with PCPs, referrals, communication with PCPs, and assistance with system barriers. Collaborative care increases treatment adherence, remission rates, quality of life, functional status, and patient satisfaction in primary care settings. **(pp. 34–36, 38)**

2. **The correct response is option C: Follow up with a nurse manager every month and a PCP every 3–6 months.**

   Collaborative psychiatric and primary care uses nurse managers to help manage chronic medical conditions such as diabetes with comorbid depression. When patients show improvement and are stable in their treatment, the number of visits to primary care and psychiatrists can decrease with close nurse manager follow-up. This allows for escalating the intensity of care as needed for severity of illness. **(p. 34)**

3. **The correct response is option B: It may improve her satisfaction with care.**

   A program where senior psychiatry residents administer both medical and psychiatric care exists at the Portland Veterans Affairs Health Care System. The patients seen by these residents reported improved satisfaction with their care. They did not have significant differences in psychiatric symptom burden, active medical problems, or screening rates for preventive health care when compared with matched patients seen by internal medicine residents and staff. The psychiatry residents reported feeling more prepared than their peers to address medical concerns and greater comfort in knowing when to refer patients for medical care. **(pp. 32–33)**

CHAPTER 5

Coronary Artery Disease

Clinical Case 1

1. **The correct response is option A: Lisinopril.**

   Lisinopril is an angiotensin-converting enzyme (ACE) inhibitor, a common first-line antihypertensive agent for treating people with diabetes. The kidneys excrete lithium, and the risk for lithium toxicity increases with the use of an ACE inhibitor. Angiotensin receptor blockers (ARBs) also act on the kidney and increase the risk for toxicity. Nearly 3% of cases of lithium toxicity are attributed to initiation of ACE inhibitors or ARBs. Psychiatrists should monitor for lithium toxicity during initiation or change in dose of ACE inhibitors or ARBs. **(p. 55)**

2. **The correct response is option B: Antiplatelet therapy.**

   Following stent placement, Ms. Jones should be treated with combination aspirin and clopidogrel or with a newer antiplatelet agent such as ticagrelor or prasugrel to prevent stent thrombosis. Length of antiplatelet therapy depends on stent type, with drug-eluting stents requiring 1 year and bare metal stents requiring at least 4 weeks. Hormone therapy is not recommended for secondary prevention of coronary artery disease (CAD). Additionally, supplementation with vitamins B_6, B_{12}, C, or E, or with folic acid or β-carotene, is not recommended. Short-acting dihydropyridine calcium channel blockers such as nifedipine may actually cause reflex tachycardia, resulting in increased myocardial demand and ischemia. A β-blocker may also be added to her regimen to reduce cardiac remodeling after myocardial infarction. **(pp. 52–54)**

3. **The correct response is option F: Answers A, B, and D.**

Ms. Jones would benefit from a number of lifestyle changes, including smoking cessation, exercise, weight loss, and improvements in her diet. A diet rich in fruits, vegetables, legumes, nuts, whole grains, and omega-3 fatty acids is recommended. Polyunsaturated fats from nuts, fish, and certain oils improve cardiovascular health, but trans fats and saturated fats should be eliminated. **(p. 52)**

Clinical Case 2

1. **The correct response is option C: 40%.**

Nearly 40% of patients with CAD have clinically significant depressive symptoms, and 20% of individuals with CAD have major depressive disorder. In contrast, only 5%–10% of persons without CAD have major depressive disorder. Depression also has a significant effect on post-myocardial infarction outcomes with higher rates of sudden cardiac death. For patients like Mr. Ames, depression screening and treatment, especially after myocardial infarction, are critical to his overall health. **(pp. 49–50)**

2. **The correct response is option F: None of the above.**

Current evidence does not support an association between use of β-blockers and the initiation or worsening of depression. Given the high comorbidity of depression and CAD, as well as worse outcomes following myocardial infarction for patients with depression, depression should not be considered a barrier to optimal medical therapy. β-Blockers are typically part of CHF management but may be held in acute CHF exacerbations. Cardioselective β-blockers such as metoprolol can be used carefully in patients with mild to moderate COPD. β-Blockers should generally be avoided in severe or decompensated COPD to prevent bronchospasm from bronchial β_2 receptor binding. Severe diabetes with recurrent hypoglycemia may be another contraindication. Overall, although the severity of the above conditions and overall clinical picture should be considered, none of these conditions is an *absolute* contraindication. **(pp. 52, 53, 55)**

3. **The correct response is option E: All of the above.**

   Takotsubo cardiomyopathy, also known as *stress cardiomyopathy*, presents as an acute coronary syndrome but occurs in the absence of occlusive CAD. The myocardial dysfunction is triggered by intense emotional or physical stress such as the death of a loved one or domestic abuse. Mental stress–induced myocardial ischemia occurs in many people with CAD and may cause coronary events at rates higher than those caused by exercise-induced ischemia. Mental stress may contribute to the pathogenesis of CAD through sympathetic activation, vagal deactivation, hypothalamic-pituitary-adrenocortical activity, and release of inflammatory mediators. **(p. 49)**

Clinical Case 3

1. **The correct response is option E: All of the above.**

   Compared with individuals without mental illness, patients with severe chronic mental illness have higher rates of all the listed modifiable risk factors and are more likely to experience higher CAD-related morbidity and mortality. The higher risk may be due to decreased access and underutilization of primary care, lower socioeconomic status, and clinical symptoms of disease (e.g., apathy, amotivation, disorganization, paranoia), which lead to poor self-care and difficulty adhering to programs designed to address lifestyle modifications. **(pp. 47–49)**

2. **The correct response is option G: Answers C and D.**

   The Framingham risk calculator is a commonly used tool in primary prevention to determine risk for myocardial infarction in the next 10 years for individuals ages 20 and older who do not have heart disease or diabetes. The following information contributes to the calculation: age, gender, total cholesterol, high-density lipoprotein cholesterol, smoking status, systolic blood pressure, and use of antihypertensive medication. Diabetes and systolic blood pressure have the greatest impact on CAD risk. Diabetes is not included in the risk calculator because it is considered a CAD equivalent. The original Framingham risk score model did not include BMI. However, the Framingham Heart Study group subsequently developed a simpler office-based nonlaboratory model that replaced lipids with BMI. The simpler model can be downloaded in Excel format at https://www.framinghamheartstudy.org/risk-functions/cardiovascular-disease/10-year-risk.php.

The ASCVD (atherosclerotic cardiovascular disease) risk assessment tool may also be used in clinical practice. **(pp. 47–48)**

3. **The correct response is option F: Answers A and D.**

BMI, blood pressure, fasting plasma glucose, and fasting lipid profile should be assessed at baseline and at regular intervals to monitor for metabolic syndrome from second-generation antipsychotic use (Table 5–1). Electrolyte measurement and a screening ECG are not among the recommended monitoring parameters. However, an ECG would be important to identify abnormalities such as QT prolongation prior to starting psychotropic medications known to alter cardiac conduction. **(pp. 56–57)**

TABLE 5–1. Baseline and ongoing monitoring for patients prescribed second-generation antipsychotics

Parameter and timing	Weight (BMI)	Waist circumference	Blood pressure	Fasting plasma glucose	Fasting lipid profile
Before prescribing second-generation antipsychotics, confirm personal and family history of obesity, diabetes mellitus, dyslipidemia, hypertension, and cardiovascular disease.					
If patient is overweight or obese, consider referral for nutrition and physical activity counseling.					
Educate patients and family members regarding signs and symptoms of diabetes mellitus.					
Baseline	X	X	X	X	X
4 weeks	X				
8 weeks	X				
12 weeks	X		X	X	X
Quarterly	X				
Annually		X	X	X	
Every 5 years					X
Treat or refer for treatment if obesity, diabetes mellitus, dyslipidemia, hypertension, or cardiovascular disease is identified.					
If parameters worsen, consider tapering or switching antipsychotic medication.					

Note. BMI = body mass index.
Source. Adapted from American Diabetes Association, American Psychiatric Association, American Association of Clinical Endocrinologists, North American Association for the Study of Obesity: "Consensus Development Conference on Antipsychotic Drugs and Obesity and Diabetes." *Diabetes Care* 27:596–601, 2004.

CHAPTER 6

Hypertension

Clinical Case 1

1. **The correct response is option C: Stage 1 hypertension.**

   Normal blood pressure is defined as less than 120/80 mmHg (Table 6–1); prehypertension is defined as blood pressure between 120/80 mmHg and 139/89 mmHg; stage 1 hypertension is defined as blood pressure between 140/90 mmHg and 159/99 mmHg; and stage 2 hypertension is defined as 160/100 mmHg or higher. In short, for systolic blood pressure, every 20 mmHg above 120 is classified into a particular stage. A diastolic blood pressure greater than 120 mmHg with end-organ damage (e.g., retinal hemorrhage, hypertensive encephalopathy) is classified as malignant hypertension, and without end-organ damage is classified as hypertensive urgency. **(pp. 65–66)**

TABLE 6–1. Diagnostic classification of blood pressure

Classification	Systolic blood pressure		Diastolic blood pressure
Normal	<120 mmHg	AND	<80 mmHg
Prehypertension	120–139 mmHg	OR	80–89 mmHg
Stage 1 hypertension	140–159 mmHg	OR	90–99 mmHg
Stage 2 hypertension	≥160 mmHg	OR	≥100 mmHg

Source. Adapted from U.S. Department of Health and Human Services: *The Seventh Report of the Joint National Committee on Prevention, Detection, Evaluation, and Treatment of High Blood Pressure.* Publ No 04-5230. Rockville, MD, National Institutes of Health, National Heart, Lung, and Blood Institute, National High Blood Pressure Education Program, August 2004. Available at: http://www.nhlbi.nih.gov/files/docs/guidelines/jnc7full.pdf.

2. **The correct response is option C: Calcium channel blocker (CCB).**

   Thiazide-type diuretics or CCBs should be used as first-line treatment of hypertension for black patients without kidney disease, whether or not they have diabetes (Figure 6–1). In this population, ACE inhibitors and ARBs are less effective and may increase the risk for stroke. For black and nonblack adults who have chronic kidney disease and hypertension, an ACE inhibitor or ARB should be first-line treatment for those with or without diabetes. Of note, β-blockers are no longer routinely used to treat hypertension but are often used for other reasons such as systolic heart failure and stable angina. **(pp. 69–70)**

3. **The correct response is option A: Essential or idiopathic hypertension.**

   All of the listed options are common causes of hypertension, but essential or idiopathic hypertension is the most common. Although most diagnoses of hypertension are categorized as essential hypertension (also termed *primary* or *idiopathic hypertension*), consideration of a broad differential diagnosis is indicated when patients are taking multiple medications with suboptimal results. **(pp. 65–66)**

4. **The correct response is option A: 2.**

   For every 20 mmHg of systolic blood pressure above 115 mmHg, there is a twofold increase in death from stroke and CAD. Hypertension is a major risk factor for cardiovascular disease, directly contributing to one-quarter of all heart attacks and one-third of all strokes. The management of hypertension decreases the risk of vascular disease, including strokes and heart attacks. **(pp. 63–64)**

Clinical Case 2

1. **The correct response is option C: 4–9 mm/Hg.**

   Engaging in aerobic activity for 30 minutes a day most days of the week would be expected to result in a 4–9 mm/Hg drop in systolic blood pressure (SBP). A weight loss of up to 20 lbs would be expected to result in a SBP reduction of 5–20 mm/Hg. Limiting alcohol consumption to no more than two drinks per day would result in a 2–4 mm/Hg reduction in SBP. **(p. 68)**

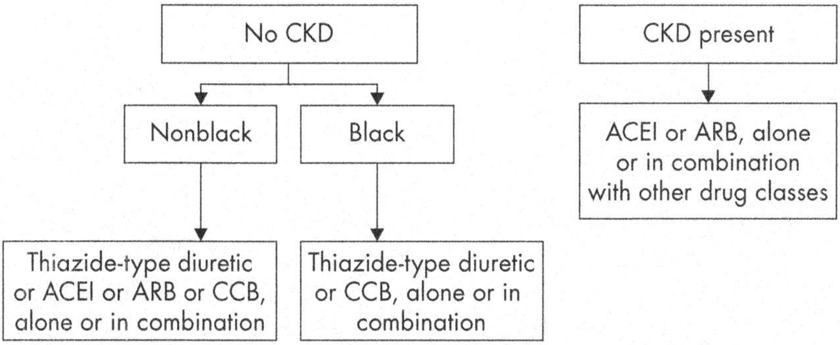

FIGURE 6–1. Treatment of hypertension, based on age, diabetes, and chronic kidney disease.

Note. ACEI = angiotensin-converting enzyme inhibitor; ARB = angiotensin receptor blocker; CCB = calcium channel blocker; CKD = chronic kidney disease.
Source. Adapted from James PA, Oparil S, Carter BL, et al.: "2014 Evidence-Based Guideline for the Management of High Blood Pressure in Adults—Report From the Panel Members Appointed to the Eighth Joint National Committee (JNC 8)." *JAMA* 311:507–520, 2014.

2. **The correct response is option B: Calcium channel blocker (CCB).**

   The recommended initial medication options for the treatment of hypertension in a white male without kidney disease are a thiazide diuretic, CCB, ACE inhibitor, or ARB (see Figure 6–1). However, treatment with a thiazide diuretic, ACE inhibitor, or ARB could complicate Mr. Neel's bipolar treatment, because lithium is renally excreted, and therefore his lithium dose may need to be reduced and his levels would have to be more closely monitored. A CCB would not affect renal function and would be the best initial choice. β-Blockers are no longer recommended as an initial treatment for hypertension unless comorbidities require otherwise. **(p. 70)**

3. **The correct response is option C: Less than 140/90 mmHg.**

   For Mr. Neel, who is younger than 60 years and has hypertension but does not have diabetes or kidney disease, the blood pressure goal is less than 140/90 (Figure 6–2). For individuals with the same medical description who are older than 60 years, the blood pressure goal is less than 150/90. For individuals who have hypertension in addition to diabetes and/or kidney disease, the goal is less than 140/90 regardless of age. **(p. 69)**

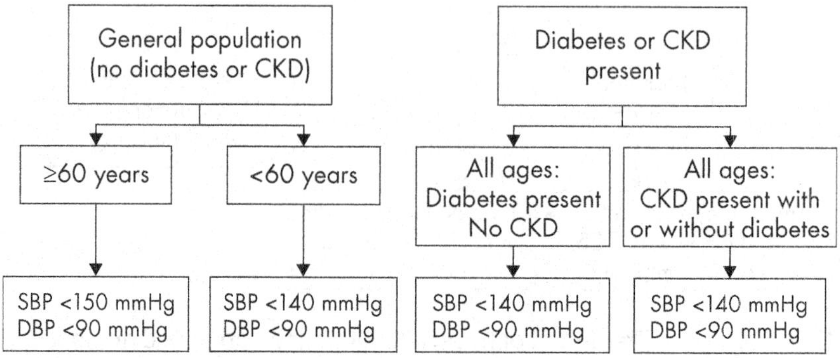

FIGURE 6–2. Treatment goals for hypertension.

Note. CKD=chronic kidney disease; DBP=diastolic blood pressure; SBP=systolic blood pressure.

Source. Adapted from Adapted from James PA, Oparil S, Carter BL, et al.: "2014 Evidence-Based Guideline for the Management of High Blood Pressure in Adults—Report From the Panel Members Appointed to the Eighth Joint National Committee (JNC 8)." *JAMA* 311:507–520, 2014.

CHAPTER 7

Dyslipidemia

Clinical Case 1

1. **The correct response is option B: 35 for men; 45 for women.**

   The USPSTF recommends screening males at average risk for dyslipidemias at age 35 and females at age 45. Individuals for whom antipsychotics are being considered should be screened for dyslipidemia before starting and every 1–3 years while taking an antipsychotic, regardless of age. **(pp. 80–81)**

2. **The correct response is option A: <20%.**

   Up to 88% of patients with schizophrenia diagnosed with dyslipidemia do not receive treatment, making it one of the most prevalent yet undertreated risk factors for cardiovascular disease (CVD) among individuals with severe mental illness. **(p. 76)**

3. **The correct response is option E: Answers A and C.**

   A lipid panel and hemoglobin A_{1c} test encompass all of the necessary blood work to establish a dyslipidemia diagnosis and establish a treatment plan. The diagnosis and treatment of dyslipidemia are now based on the assessment of an individual's risk for atherosclerotic CVD. Components of the risk assessment include gender, age, race, total cholesterol, high-density lipoprotein (HDL) cholesterol, systolic blood pressure, treatment for hypertension, diabetes status, and current smoking status. The decision to treat and the intensity of treatment are no longer based on low-density lipoprotein (LDL) cholesterol alone. However, if the initial screening LDL is very high (≥190), a high-intensity statin would be indicated and a workup for secondary causes of dyslipidemia should be pursued (Table 7–1). If the initial LDL is <190, the treatment intensity would be based on atherosclerotic CVD risk assessment rather than LDL. **(pp. 78–80)**

4. **The correct response is option C: Get a nonfasting lipid panel now.**

   Instructing Mr. Helms to get a nonfasting lipid panel today, while he is already at the clinic, has the greatest chance for success. Non-HDL cholesterol (total cholesterol minus HDL cholesterol) may be more reliable than LDL as an indicator of CVD risk and can be calculated without regard to fasting status. **(p. 77)**

Clinical Case 2

1. **The correct response is option D: Statin medication.**

   Because of their proven efficacy, ease of use, and relatively safe profiles, statin medications are the first choice and are well tolerated in patients. Alternative drug therapies have not conclusively been shown to reduce the rate of stroke or myocardial infarction. Individuals ages 40–75 years without clinical atherosclerotic CVD or diabetes and an estimated 10-year atherosclerotic CVD risk greater than or equal to 7.5% should be treated with a moderate- to high-intensity statin. This patient has a 10-year atherosclerotic CVD risk of 8.5%, qualifying her for statin treatment. **(pp. 81, 82, 87)**

2. **The correct response is option D: Non-HDL cholesterol.**

   Non-HDL cholesterol should be used. The patient provided a blood sample for a nonfasting lipid panel. The calculated LDL is incorrectly low because of the elevated triglyceride level from the nonfasting sample. Non-HDL cholesterol, calculated by subtracting HDL from the total cholesterol, is significantly elevated at 210 mg/dL. Non-HDL cholesterol levels can be roughly correlated to LDL levels by subtracting 30. Thus, a non-HDL cholesterol level of 210 mg/dL would be equivalent to an LDL level of 180 mg/dL. With an LDL level of 180 mg/dL, the decision to treat with a statin would be based on the 10-year atherosclerotic CVD risk assessment because only an LDL level of at least 190

TABLE 7–1. Four clinical classes of statin eligibility

Clinical characteristic	Type of prevention[a]	Applicable age range	Preferred statin intensity	Potential actions
Clinical presence of CVD	Secondary	21–75	High	—
Serum LDL ≥190 mg/dL[b]	Primary	21–75	High	Work up potential secondary causes[c]
Type 2 diabetes[d]	Primary	40–75	Moderate to high	—
10-year risk >7.5%[d]	Primary	40–75	Moderate	—

Note. CVD = cardiovascular disease; LDL = low-density lipoprotein.
[a]Primary prevention takes place when there is no clinical evidence of disease. Secondary prevention applies to therapies in place after the clinical presence of disease.
[b]Individuals with non-high-density lipoprotein (HDL) cholesterol (total cholesterol – HDL cholesterol) greater than 220 mg/dL also fall into this category.
[c]Potential secondary causes.
[d]These recommendations apply to individuals with LDL cholesterol values of 70–189 mg/dL.
Source. Adapted from Stone NJ, Robinson JG, Lichtenstein AH, et al.: "2013 ACC/AHA Guideline on Treatment of Blood Cholesterol to Reduce Atherosclerotic Cardiovascular Risk in Adults: A Report of the American College of Cardiology/American Heart Association Task Force on Practice Guidelines." *Journal of the American College of Cardiology* 63(25, pt B):2889–2934, 2014.

automatically qualifies a patient for high-intensity statin treatment without the risk assessment. **(pp. 79–80)**

3. **The correct response is option B: Begin a moderate- to high-intensity statin.**

With a non-HDL cholesterol level of 210 mg/dL (roughly equivalent to an LDL of 180 mg/dL), Ms. Roberts does not immediately qualify for a high-intensity statin. A non-HDL level of 220 mg/dL would qualify. Ms. Roberts has a hemoglobin A_{1c} value of 5.5 and therefore does not qualify for moderate- to high-dose statin therapy based on diabetes. The next step is to calculate her 10-year atherosclerotic CVD risk using an online calculator. Her calculated 10-year atherosclerotic CVD risk is 8.5%. A risk greater than 7.5% qualifies for primary prevention of atherosclerotic CVD with a moderate- to high-intensity statin. The American College of Cardiology provides free iPhone, Android, or Web-based apps to quickly calculate the risk scores and recommendations for intensity of treatment. These resources can be accessed at http://www.cardiosource.org/science-and-quality/practice-guidelines-and-quality-standards/2013-prevention-guideline-tools.aspx. **(p. 78)**

Clinical Case 3

1. **The correct response is option C: Secondary causes of hyperlipidemia.**

   Mr. Lewis should be evaluated for secondary causes of hyperlipidemia because his LDL is greater than 190 (see Table 7–2 for leading secondary causes of severely elevated blood cholesterol). Measurement of waist circumference provides additional cardiovascular risk information but is not necessary before selecting a treatment. Skinfold thickness assessment is valuable in the evaluation of malnutrition but has limited utility in the management of dyslipidemia. A hemoglobin A_{1c} test was already ordered; therefore, a fasting glucose measurement would be redundant and provide less information. **(pp. 87–88)**

2. **The correct response is option A: An antipsychotic that has lower risk of metabolic syndrome.**

   Mr. Lewis has been unsuccessful with dietary and lifestyle modifications to control his cholesterol. He should continue to increase his physical activity but also needs to start an additional treatment modality. His 10-year atherosclerotic CVD risk is 27.0%, qualifying him for high-intensity statin treatment. However, he is taking an antipsychotic with high risk of metabolic syndrome and should be receive a trial of a more weight-neutral antipsychotic (e.g., perphenazine or haloperidol) before a statin is started. **(p. 81)**

3. **The correct response is option D: Answer B or C.**

   Because Mr. Lewis's 10-year atherosclerotic CVD risk is 27.0%, he should be started on a high-intensity statin. Both atorvastatin and rosuvastatin are high-potency statins used for high-intensity treatment. Pravastatin is a relatively weak statin and is used for low- to moderate-intensity treatment. Should the patient experience intolerable side effects while taking atorvastatin or rosuvastatin, pravastatin would be a good choice because it is well tolerated and has few drug-drug interactions. **(pp. 86, 88–90)**

TABLE 7–2. Leading secondary causes of severely elevated blood cholesterol

Secondary cause	Details
Disease/medical/genetic	Diabetes mellitus
	Hypothyroidism
	Chronic kidney disease
	Nephropathy, proteinuria
	Familial (genetic) hyperlipidemia
	Pregnancy[a]
Substance use	Excessive alcohol intake
Medications	Estrogen
	HIV antiretroviral therapy
	Antipsychotic medications
	Steroids, immunosuppressants
	Drug-drug interactions limiting statin efficacy
Diet	Extreme obesity
	High saturated and trans fat intake

[a]Pregnancy and lactation are contraindications to statin therapies.

Source. Adapted from Stone NJ, Robinson JG, Lichtenstein AH, et al.: "2013 ACC/AHA Guideline on the Treatment of Blood Cholesterol to Reduce Atherosclerotic Cardiovascular Risk in Adults: A Report of the American College of Cardiology/American Heart Association Task Force on Practice Guidelines." *Journal of the American College of Cardiology* 63(25, pt B):2889–2934, 2014; Vodnala D, Rubenfire M, Brook RD: "Secondary Causes of Dyslipidemia." *American Journal of Cardiology* 110:823–825, 2012.

CHAPTER 8

Tobacco Dependence

Clinical Case 1

1. **The correct response is option D: All of the above.**

   Genetic predisposition through abnormal cholinergic mechanisms and nicotinic receptors may lead to greater reward from nicotine, which ameliorates some of the deficits in sensory processing, attention, cognition, and mood. Tobacco smoke may inhibit monoamine oxidase, leading to an antidepressant effect. Historically, smoking in treatment facilities is common and sometimes encouraged (by using cigarettes as behavioral rewards). **(p. 96)**

2. **The correct response is option D: Rates have not declined.**

   The fact that rates have not declined may partially explain why individuals with severe mental illness die an average of 25 years earlier than individuals without mental illness. Psychiatrists are well positioned to use psychotherapy skills, mainly in the form of cognitive-behavioral therapy and motivational interviewing, to help patients stop smoking. **(p. 96)**

3. **The correct response is option C: Combined treatment with medications and psychosocial treatments.**

   Both smoking cessation medications and psychosocial treatments are effective independently; however, combined treatment is superior to either treatment alone. There is no evidence showing psychodynamic psychotherapy to be beneficial in smoking cessation. **(p. 100)**

4. **The correct response is option D: Varenicline.**

Varenicline is efficacious and least likely to precipitate a manic episode (Table 8–1). It is associated with worsened depression and suicidal ideation but is usually well tolerated. Nortriptyline and bupropion are riskier options because of the potential for precipitating a manic episode. Nicotine replacement is unlikely to worsen psychiatric symptoms, but associated quit rates are relatively modest. **(pp. 100, 102–103)**

Clinical Case 2

1. **The correct response is option D: Motivational interviewing.**

This is an example of motivational interviewing. By being less directive and letting the patient explore her own motivations for and against smoking, the mental health provider facilitates the development of motivation necessary for the patient to stop smoking. Problem solving, a component of supportive therapy, can be beneficial in overcoming relapses. Psychoeducation and cognitive-behavioral therapy are additional therapeutic modalities with proven effectiveness. **(pp. 99, 101)**

2. **The correct response is option C: 10 lbs.**

A meta-analysis published in 2012 showed that individuals gained an average of 10.4 lbs over 12 months following smoking cessation. Most of the weight gain occurred within the first 3 months. (Aubin HJ, Farley A, Lycett D, et al.: Weight gain in smokers after quitting cigarettes: meta-analysis. BMJ Jul 10, 345:e4439) **(pp. 98–99)**

3. **The correct response is option B: Bupropion.**

Bupropion would complement Mrs. Peter's antidepressant regimen, is effective for smoking cessation, and would be unlikely to contribute to further weight gain. Nortriptyline would potentially help with her depressive symptoms; however, less evidence supports its use in smoking cessation, and it may contribute to weight gain. Varenicline would not help with her depressive symptoms. Nicotine replacement would help with smoking cessation but would not have an impact on her mood. **(pp. 100, 102–105)**

TABLE 8–1. Smoking cessation medications

Drug	Daily dosage	Treatment duration	Potential side effects
First-line treatments			
Nicotine replacement therapy			
Transdermal 24-hour patch (over the counter)	21 mg/day to start 7- and 14-mg patches for tapering dosage	8–12 weeks	Skin irritation, insomnia
Polacrilex (gum), 2- or 4-mg piece (over the counter)	1 piece/hour (<24 pieces/day)	8–12 weeks	Mouth irritation, sore jaw, dyspepsia, hiccups
Lozenge (over the counter)	2- or 4-mg dose (see dosage formula and titration schedule in package)	12 weeks	Hiccups, nausea, heartburn
Vapor inhaler (prescription only)	6–16 cartridges/day (delivers 4 mg/cartridge)	3–6 months	Mouth and throat irritation
Nasal spray (prescription only)	1–2 doses/hour; dose = 1 mg (0.5 mg per nostril); maximum dosage 40 mg/day	3–6 months	Nasal irritation, sneezing, cough, tearing eyes
Approved non-nicotine medications			
Bupropion (sustained release)	150 mg/day for 3 days, then 150 mg bid; start 1 week before quit date	7–12 weeks; up to 6 months to maintain abstinence	Insomnia, dry mouth, neuropsychiatric symptoms including depression, suicidal thoughts, agitation *Contraindications:* seizures, eating disorders
Varenicline	0.5 mg/day for 3 days, then 0.5 mg bid for 4 days, then 1 mg bid for 3 months; start 1 week before quit date	12–24 weeks	Nausea, headache, insomnia, vivid dreams, neuropsychiatric symptoms including depression, suicidal thoughts, agitation

TABLE 8–1. Smoking cessation medications *(continued)*

Drug	Daily dosage	Treatment duration	Potential side effects
Second-line treatments[a]			
Nortriptyline	75–100 mg/day; start 10–28 days prior to quit date at 25 mg/day and increase as tolerated	12 weeks	Dry mouth, sedation, dizziness, suicidal thoughts
Clonidine		3–10 weeks	Dry mouth, sedation, dizziness
Combination nicotine replacement therapy			

[a]Recommended in the Clinical Practice Guideline (Fiore et al. 2008) but not approved for this indication by the U.S. Food and Drug Administration. Fiore MC, Jaen CR, Baker TB, et al.: *Treating Tobacco Use and Dependence: 2008 Update.* Clinical Practice Guideline. Rockville, MD, U.S. Department of Health and Human Services Public Health Service, 2008.

CHAPTER 9

Chronic Obstructive Pulmonary Disease

Clinical Case 1

1. **The correct response is option C: Spiromerty.**

   Classic symptoms and history can be strongly suggestive of chronic obstructive pulmonary disease (COPD) (Figure 9–1), but spirometry is the gold standard for diagnosing COPD. Physical examination is not sensitive for diagnosing COPD because many of the classic findings are present only with severe disease. Imaging studies can support clinical suspicion for COPD but are not used to make the diagnosis. **(pp. 115–116)**

2. **The correct response is option A: He has COPD.**

   A diagnosis of COPD is confirmed with an FEV_1/FVC ratio less than 0.7 and an FEV1 less than 80% (Figure 9–2). With an FEV_1/FVC ratio of 0.6 and an FEV_1 of 72%, the criteria for COPD are met for this patient. Imaging studies are not needed for the diagnosis of COPD. **(p. 117)**

3. **The correct response is option C: Smoking cessation.**

   The long-term benefits of smoking cessation in the treatment of COPD are well documented. Following cessation there is a substantial improvement in cough, expectoration, breathlessness, and wheezing. The

Risk factors

- Smoking (number of pack-years smoked = packs of cigarettes per day × the number of years)
- Asthma
- Long-term exposure to aerosolized irritants (e.g., chemical dusts, fumes, vapors)
- Family history of lung disease

Symptoms

- Progressive and intermittent dyspnea
- Cough, usually worse in the mornings and productive of small amount of colorless sputum
- Wheezing, particularly during exertion and exacerbations
- Recurrent upper respiratory infections

Physical exam (findings are generally present only with severe disease)

- Pursed-lip breathing
- Cyanosis
- Barrel chest (hyperinflation)
- Hyperresonance on percussion
- Use of accessory respiratory muscles and/or intercostal retractions (Hoover's sign)
- Prolonged expiratory phase
- Decreased intensity of breath and heart sounds
- Wheezing during slow or forced breathing
- Mild dependent edema
- Digital clubbing

FIGURE 9–1. History and physical findings in chronic obstructive pulmonary disease.

remaining response options are important components in the management of COPD, but none of them have as much impact as smoking cessation. **(pp. 118–119)**

4. **The correct response is option D: Answers B and C.**

Clozapine toxicity and weight gain are potential adverse effects of smoking cessation. Smoking increases the metabolism of some antipsychotics including clozapine. As Mr. Kelso stops smoking, clozapine may accumulate, thereby causing toxicity. Clozapine levels should be measured before and after smoking cessation to determine whether dosing adjustments need to be made. There is typically some weight gain following smoking cessation; however, the health benefits exceed the problems associated with modest weight gain. Several studies have shown that psychiatric symptoms do not worsen when patients participate in smoking cessation treatment. **(pp. 97–99, 105, 120)**

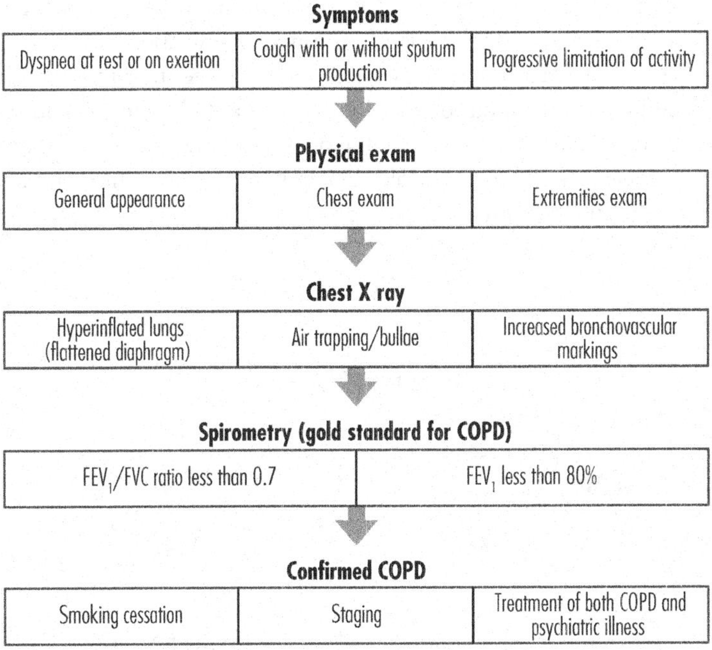

FIGURE 9–2. Clinical assessment for chronic obstructive pulmonary disease (COPD).

Note. FEV_1 = forced expiratory volume after 1 second; FVC = forced vital capacity.

Clinical Case 2

1. **The correct response is option D: Referral to a primary care provider.**

   Referral to her primary care physician to start an inhaled corticosteroid would be the next step in managing symptomatic COPD not adequately treated by a long-acting inhaled β_2-agonist and short-acting bronchodilators. Lorazepam and codeine have respiratory depressing effects and should be avoided if possible. Because the patient's cough appears to be the primary issue, increasing her antipsychotic will not likely improve the situation. **(pp. 119–121)**

2. **The correct response is option C: Call the group home operator to verify compliance.**

   Verification of compliance with her increasingly complex medication regimen would be the most appropriate next step. Enlisting staff at her group home to assist with medications could be helpful. Also, simply discussing the patient's understanding of her medication regimen may improve compliance. Complex medication regimens should be simplified as much as possible among patients with serious mental illness. The addition of a long-acting anticholinergic and referral to a pulmonologist are potential next steps that the patient's primary care provider may undertake. Theophylline is an option, but it is not a first-line recommendation for escalation of therapy (Figure 9–3). **(pp. 118–119)**

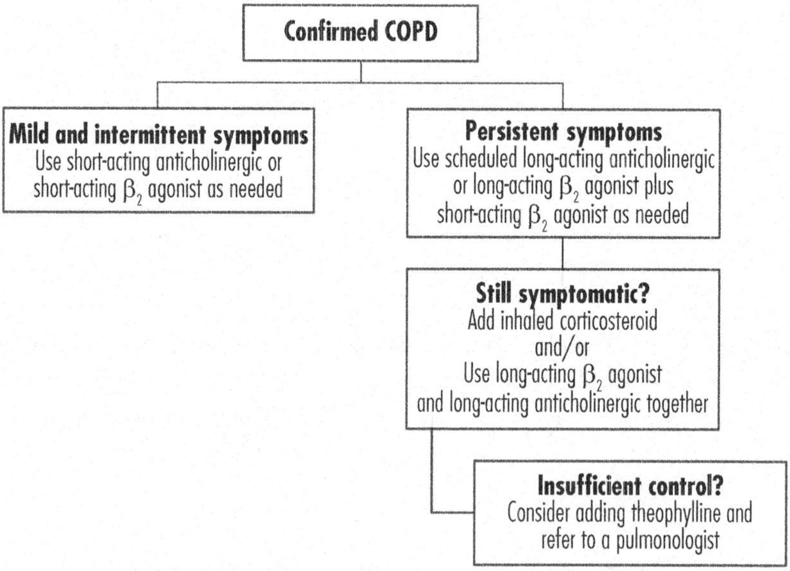

FIGURE 9–3. Algorithm for pharmacological management of chronic obstructive pulmonary disease (COPD) in an ambulatory setting.

Source. Adapted from Global Initiative for Chronic Obstructive Lung *Disease: Global Strategy for the Diagnosis, Management, and Prevention of Chronic Obstructive Pulmonary Disease.* Vancouver, WA, Global Initiative for Chronic Obstructive Lung Disease, 2013.

3. **The correct response is option E: Answers C and D.**

The pneumococcal and influenza vaccinations are of particular benefit in patients with COPD. **(p. 121)**

CHAPTER 10

Diabetes

Clinical Case 1

1. **The correct response is option C: Start an SSRI and check hemoglobin A_{1c} (HbA_{1c}).**

   This patient has multiple risk factors for developing diabetes, including family history, elevated body mass index (BMI), and depression. Patients over age 45 years or with a BMI of at least 25 plus one or more risk factors require annual screening for diabetes. Patients with depression are at increased risk for developing diabetes, even when BMI, hypertension, and family history are controlled for. Tricyclic antidepressants (e.g., imipramine) are associated with weight gain and hyperglycemia and therefore would not be appropriate in a patient who is overweight with a BMI of 29.3. Ms. Amber's blood pressure is at goal for her age (<140/90 mmHg), and she should not start taking an antihypertensive. A selective serotonin reuptake inhibitor (SSRI) may be a good choice; fluoxetine and sertraline have been associated with improved glycemic control, whereas paroxetine and mirtazapine have been associated with weight gain. **(pp. 129, 131, 137)**

2. **The correct response is option D: Prediabetes.**

   Prediabetes is diagnosed when one of the following criteria is met: an HbA_{1c} value of 5.7%–6.4%, a fasting glucose level of 100–125 mg/dL, or a 2-hour plasma glucose of 140–199 mg/dL during an oral glucose tolerance test. An HbA_{1c} is often easiest to check because it does not require fasting. Type 2 diabetes is a result of impaired insulin sensitivity and liver gluconeogenesis, whereas type 1 diabetes results from impaired insulin production in the pancreas. Type 1 and type 2 diabetes are differentiated by underlying pathophysiology, not blood glucose levels, age, or HbA_{1c} value. An HbA_{1c} value greater than or equal to 6.5% is consistent with a diagnosis of diabetes. **(pp. 128, 130–131)**

Diagnosis of Diabetes

The diagnosis of diabetes requires one of the following:

- Fasting blood glucose of > 126 mg/dL on 2 separate days
- Symptoms of hyperglycemia plus a random plasma glucose of ≥200 mg/dL
- Two-hour plasma glucose of ≥200 mg/dL during an oral glucose tolerance test (OGTT), with results duplicated on a separate day
- HbA_{1c} of ≥6.5%

Prediabetes can be identified with the same tests used to diagnose diabetes and is defined as follows:

- Fasting blood glucose of 100–125 mg/dL
- Two-hour plasma glucose of 140–199 mg/dL during an OGTT
- HbA_{1c} of 5.7%–6.4%

Symptoms of prediabetes may include thirst, frequent urination, increased appetite, fatigue, frequent infections, slow healing of cuts or wounds, blurry vision, and numbness or tingling in extremities. Patients whose testing is consistent with prediabetes should be monitored yearly.

A simple screening and diagnostic test for diabetes is the HbA_{1c} test. The use of HbA_{1c} values for diagnosis was recently updated by the American Diabetes Association in 2014 to improve the diagnostic rate for diabetes. The fact that neither fasting nor the OGTT is required for the HbA_{1c} test is especially relevant for patients with mental illness, because it is often challenging to obtain fasting test results or to perform the OGTT. The HbA_{1c} value gives a sense of average blood glucose levels in the past 120 days.

Screening for diabetes should be considered in all adults over age 45 or those who are overweight (BMI≥25) with one or more of the following risk factors:

- Physical inactivity
- First-degree relative with diabetes
- High-risk race/ethnicity (e.g., African American, Latino, Native American, Asian American, Pacific Islander)

- Having delivered a baby weighing more than 4 kg (9 lb), or having been diagnosed with gestational diabetes mellitus
- Hypertension (having blood pressure of ≥140/90 mmHg, or taking an antihypertensive)
- A high-density lipoprotein cholesterol level of <35 mg/dL and/or a triglyceride level of >250 mg/dL
- Polycystic ovary syndrome (in women)
- HbA_{1c} of ≥5.7%, impaired glucose tolerance, or impaired fasting glucose on previous testing
- Other clinical conditions associated with insulin resistance (e.g., severe obesity, acanthosis nigricans)
- History of cardiovascular disease

Clinical Case 2

1. **The correct response is option C: Increase metformin to 1,000 mg bid and check HbA_{1c} every 3 months.**

   The patient is currently taking a low dose of metformin with inadequate control of his diabetes, as indicated by his most recent HbA_{1c} value of 7.9%. His metformin dose should be adjusted to target an HbA_{1c} value of less than 7.0%. Metformin should not be dosed above 2,000 mg/day. HbA_{1c} should be checked every 3 months if medications are being adjusted or if blood sugars are poorly controlled. In patients with glycemic control at goal, HbA_{1c} can be checked every 6–12 months. **(p. 133)**

2. **The correct response is option E: All of the above.**

   Patients with diabetes require annual screening for diabetic retinopathy, diabetic nephropathy, and peripheral neuropathy. Thus, they should have a dilated eye examination, urine studies (urine albumin and creatinine to check albumin-to-creatinine ratio), basic metabolic panel to check creatinine, and a diabetic foot examination every year, regardless of age and HbA_{1c} value, Lipid panels should also be checked yearly in all patients with diabetes (Table 10–1). **(pp. 135–136)**

3. **The correct response is option C: Start lisinopril 10 mg/day to target a blood pressure of <140/90 mmHg.**

   The goal blood pressure for patients with diabetes (regardless of age) is less than 140/90. Mr. Beal's blood pressure has been consistently

TABLE 10–1. Blood pressure and lipid goals

Measure	Goal
Blood pressure	
Systolic	<140 mmHg
Diastolic	<90 mmHg
Fasting lipid panel	
Total	<200 mg/dL
Triglycerides	<150 mg/dL
Low-density lipoprotein	<100 mg/dL[a]
High-density lipoprotein	>40 mg/dL (men); >50 mg/dL (women)

[a]Low-density lipoprotein goal is <70 mg/dL among patients with cardiovascular disease.

elevated, so it is appropriate to start medication. First-line treatment for hypertension in diabetic patients is either an angiotensin-converting enzyme (ACE) inhibitor, such as lisinopril, or an angiotensin II receptor blocker (ARB). In addition to lowering blood pressure, ACE inhibitors and ARBs protect against kidney damage and slow progression of diabetic kidney disease. Many patients will require more than one agent to control their blood pressure. **(pp. 133–135)**

Clinical Case 3

1. **The correct response is option B: Olanzapine can increase risk for diabetes.**

   Ms. Cathol has had significant weight gain in the last year, which is generally defined as a weight gain of at least 7% from baseline. Of the second-generation antipsychotics (SGAs), clozapine and olanzapine are the most likely to cause weight gain and increase the risk of diabetes. She is experiencing polyuria and polydipsia, which are common when blood glucose levels are elevated. Weight loss can reduce hyperglycemia and reduce risk for developing diabetes and therefore is important to discuss with all patients taking SGAs. **(pp. 137–138)**

2. **The correct response is option D: All of the above.**

   It is appropriate to consider all of the above interventions. Medications that cause weight gain result in increased risk for development of diabetes. Switching medications should be considered in any patient who gains more than 5% of his or her baseline weight. Of the SGAs, lurasidone, ziprasidone, and aripiprazole have the lowest associated risk for diabetes and weight gain. Lifestyle modifications to promote weight loss (e.g., diet and exercise) are first-line therapies in preventing and managing all patients with diabetes. The addition of metformin can mitigate weight gain associated with SGAs and prevent progression to diabetes in patients with prediabetes. **(pp. 132, 133, 137–138, 176)**

CHAPTER 11

Obesity

Clinical Case 1

1. **The correct response is option C: As a class, antipsychotics are associated with more weight gain than mood stabilizers or antidepressants.**

   Antipsychotics, as a group, are associated with more weight gain than antidepressants or mood stabilizers. In general, first-generation antipsychotics have less associated weight gain and a better metabolic profile than second-generation antipsychotics (SGAs). Of the SGAs, both olanzapine and clozapine are associated with the most weight gain, whereas ziprasidone, aripiprazole, and lurasidone have less effect on weight (although comparative studies are lacking). It is estimated that 36% of adults are obese, as defined by a BMI of 30 or more (Table 11–1). The prevalence of obesity in patients with serious mental illness is 1.5–2.0 times higher than in the general population. Obesity is associated with multiple health conditions, including type 2 diabetes, cardiovascular disease, and hypertension. **(pp. 143–147, 176)**

2. **The correct response is option D: Waist circumference annually and BMI at regular intervals.**

   Because SGAs are associated with significant weight gain, there are now guidelines for monitoring and screening for obesity in these patients. Prior to starting an SGA, providers should calculate BMI, measure waist circumference, and assess personal and family history of obe-

TABLE 11–1. Weight classifications for adults

	Body mass index
Underweight	<18.5
Normal weight	18.5–24.9
Overweight	25.0–29.9
Grade I obesity	30.0–34.9
Grade II obesity	35.0–39.9
Grade III obesity	≥40

Source. Adapted from National Heart, Lung, and Blood Institute; Obesity Education Initiative Expert Panel on the Identification, Evaluation, and Treatment of Obesity in Adults: *Clinical Guidelines on the Identification, Evaluation, and Treatment of Overweight and Obesity in Adults.* Bethesda, MD, National Heart, Lung, and Blood Institute, 1998.

sity. BMI should then be checked after starting an SGA at weeks 4, 8, and 12, and then quarterly. If BMI is stable, it can then be followed annually. Waist circumference and personal/family history should be monitored annually. Abnormal waist circumference is ≥35 inches in women and ≥40 inches in men. **(pp. 147, 149–150)**

3. **The correct response is option A: Recommend reducing caloric intake by 500–1,000 calories per day.**

The first step in addressing weight gain in patients with mental illness is to limit medications that are associated with increases in weight. Lifestyle interventions to promote weight loss should also be part of any prevention or treatment plan. Weight loss is achieved by creating a calorie deficit, either by exercising and/or reducing caloric intake. Decreasing caloric intake by 500–1,000 calories per day over 6 months will result in approximately a 10% reduction in baseline weight. The type of diet, such as a low-fat or low-carbohydrate diet, is not as important for weight loss as is the absolute reduction of caloric intake. Thus, low-calorie diets can be tailored to patient preference and availability. Bariatric surgery is an option in people with severe mental illness but is not recommended unless the individual has either a BMI of 40 or greater or a BMI of 35 and comorbidities such as diabetes or sleep apnea. Although exercise is important in creating a calorie deficit, walking 30 minutes/day 5 days a week at 4 miles/hour is recommended for maintaining weight, but is not enough to lose weight. Thus, patients who want to lose weight need to exercise more. Dietary education and cognitive-behavioral interventions, such as self-monitoring and behavior replacement, are also helpful in achieving weight loss, and should be utilized where available. **(pp. 151–153, 155, 171)**

Clinical Case 2

1. **The correct response is option D: Both A and C.**

   Obese patients are at increased risk for many chronic diseases, including type 2 diabetes, nonalcoholic fatty liver disease, cardiovascular disease, and hyperlipidemia (Table 11–2). Thus, it is important to evaluate for treatable comorbidities in obese patients. Because hypothyroidism can lead to weight gain, thyroid-stimulating hormone (TSH) should also be checked. Mirtazapine and paroxetine are both associated with weight gain, and neither would be the best choice for this patient's depression. It is also important to discuss past attempts at weight loss and reasons for weight gain. This will help the provider and the patient understand barriers and set specific goals. **(pp. 144, 147)**

2. **The correct response is option A: Metformin.**

   Mr. Tatum has diabetes, based on a hemoglobin A_{1c} value of at least 6.5%. Lifestyle modifications and metformin are typically first-line therapy in treating diabetes. Metformin lowers blood glucose by reducing hepatic gluconeogenesis and increasing insulin sensitivity. It can also promote weight loss and limit weight gain in patients taking SGAs. Although topiramate is associated with weight loss, this patient also has hyperglycemia, and metformin would be a better choice. Side effects of topiramate include somnolence and dizziness and may worsen his feelings of lethargy and fatigue. Oral agents would be first-line treatment for him (Table 11–3), and insulin would not be started unless he fails to control his diabetes by taking the oral medications alone. **(pp. 131, 138, 153, 155, 166, 168)**

3. **The correct response is option A: Hypoglycemia.**

   Gastrointestinal complaints, such as nausea, vomiting, and diarrhea, as well as metallic taste, are among the most common side effects of metformin. To minimize side effects, providers should start metformin at a low dose (500 mg bid) and then titrate as tolerated to effect. Taking it with food can also minimize the gastrointestinal side effects.

TABLE 11–2. Health conditions associated with obesity

Endocrine	Diabetes Dyslipidemia
Cardiovascular	Hypertension Coronary artery disease Stroke
Cancer	Colorectal Breast Endometrial
Gastrointestinal	Gastroesophageal reflux disease Cholelithiasis Fatty liver disease
Renal	Nephrolithiasis
Reproductive	Infertility, pregnancy complications Polycystic ovary syndrome Erectile dysfunction
Pulmonary	Obstructive sleep apnea
Musculoskeletal	Osteoarthritis Low back pain

Source. Adapted from Tsai AG, Wadden TA: "In the Clinic: Obesity." *Annals of Internal Medicine* 159:ITC3-1–ITC3-15; quiz ITC3-16, 2013.

Unlike other oral hyperglycemic agents (e.g., sulfonylureas), metformin as a monotherapy does not cause hypoglycemia and is therefore safe in patients who have low-normal blood glucose levels. It is important to remember that metformin carries a black box warning for metabolic acidosis, although its incidence is very low. Patients who have impaired renal function are at increased risk for metabolic acidosis, and kidney function should thus be monitored in patients using metformin. Use is contraindicated in patients with a glomerular filtration rate of less than 30 mL/minute. **(pp. 133, 134, 170)**

4. **The correct response is option D: Antihistamines.**

It is important to look at a patient's entire medication list and to minimize the number of obesity-related medications when possible. Numerous classes of medications are associated with weight gain, including glucocorticoids, antihistamines, diabetes medications (not including metformin), hormonal agents, β-blockers and α-blockers. Glucocorticoids and SGAs are associated with the greatest weight gain. **(p. 148)**

TABLE 11–3. Oral diabetic agents

Class	Agent	Comments
Biguanides	Metformin (Glucophage, Riomet cherry-flavored liquid) Metformin ER (Fortamet, Glumetza, Glucophage XR)	No hypoglycemia GI side effects Rare lactic acidosis Contraindicated in renal insufficiency (GFR < 30) Vitamin B_{12} deficiency
Sulfonylureas	Glipizide (Glucotrol, Glucotrol XL) Glimepiride (Amaryl) Glyburide (DiaBeta, Micronase)	Hypoglycemia Weight gain
Thiazolidinediones/glitazones	Pioglitazone (Actos)	Weight gain Heart failure Rare hepatotoxicity
Dipeptidyl peptidase–4 inhibitors	Sitagliptin (Januvia) Saxagliptin (Onglyza)	Modest effect on HbA_{1c} levels No hypoglycemia, urticaria, angioedema Small risk of pancreatitis
α-Glucosidase inhibitors	Acarbose (Precose) Miglitol (Glyset)	Modest effect on HbA_{1c} levels GI side effects
Oral β-cell stimulators	Repaglinide (Prandin) Nateglinide (Starlix)	Hypoglycemia Weight gain Short half-life

Note. ER = extended release; GFR = glomerular filtration rate; GI = gastrointestinal; HbA_{1c} = hemoglobin A_{1c}; XL = extended release; XR = extended release.

CHAPTER 12

Metabolic Syndrome

Clinical Case 1

1. **The correct response is option C: Elevated LDL.**

   Metabolic syndrome is a constellation of findings that increases a patient's risk for cardiovascular disease. A diagnosis of metabolic syndrome is made when three of the criteria shown in Table 12–1 are met. Mrs. Seits's results meet three of the criteria for metabolic syndrome: hypertriglyceridemia, low high-density lipoprotein (HDL), and impaired fasting glucose. Although this patient's low-density lipoprotein (LDL) is high, LDL is not a criterion for metabolic syndrome. It is important to remember that weight gain is the biggest risk factor for developing metabolic syndrome. It is estimated that 60% of patients with schizophrenia also have metabolic syndrome. **(pp. 161–163, 165)**

2. **The correct response is option B: Simvastatin 40 mg/day.**

   This patient has dyslipidemia and should be treated with a 3-hydroxy-3-methylglutaryl–coenzyme A (HMG-CoA) reductase inhibitor, or statin. Guidelines for appropriate initiation and choice of statins are based on the presence of cardiovascular risk factors, lipid levels, and age. Because this patient is over age 21 and has an LDL above 190 mg/dL, a statin should be initiated to reduce risk for cardiovascular disease. Although her hemoglobin A_{1c} is above goal, her metformin dose should be increased prior to adding insulin. Because her blood pressure is at goal (<140/90 mmHg) and she is already taking an angiotensin-

TABLE 12–1. Metabolic syndrome: diagnostic criteria

Three of the following criteria:

Abdominal obesity	Men: waist circumference ≥ 40 in. (102 cm) Women: waist circumference ≥ 35 in. (88 cm)
Hypertriglyceridemia	Serum TG ≥ 150 mg/dL
Low HDL cholesterol	Men: serum HDL < 40 mg/dL Women: serum HDL < 50 mg/dL
Elevated blood pressure	BP ≥ 130/85 mmHg Or medication for HTN
Impaired fasting glucose	Fasting BG ≥ 100[a] Or medication for diabetes

Note. BG = blood glucose; BP = blood pressure; HDL = high-density lipoprotein; HTN = hypertension; TG = triglycerides.

[a]Hemoglobin A_{1c} (HbA_{1c}) ≥ 6.5% is now used for the diagnosis of diabetes. HbA_{1c} ≥ 5.7% has a 91% specificity for impaired fasting glucose (BG ≥ 100 mg/dL) (American Diabetes Association: "Diagnosis and Classification of Diabetes Mellitus." *Diabetes Care* 33 (suppl 1):S62–S69, 2010).

Source. Adapted from Alberti KG, Zimmet P, Shaw J: "Metabolic Syndrome—A New Worldwide Definition: A Consensus Statement From the International Diabetes Federation. *Diabetic Medicine* 23:469–480, 2006; Expert Panel on Detection, Evaluation, and Treatment of High Blood Cholesterol in Adults: "Executive Summary of the Third Report of the National Cholesterol Education Program (NCEP) (Adult Treatment Panel III)." *JAMA* 285:2486–2497, 2001.

converting enzyme inhibitor (ACE) inhibitor, an angiotensin II receptor blocker (ARB) such as losartan need not be added. Weight loss may be improved with optimization of metformin dose, which would be more appropriate than starting topiramate. **(pp. 166, 168, 172)**

3. **The correct response is option A: BMI, blood pressure, lipid panel, and fasting glucose.**

Patients taking second-generation antipsychotics (SGAs) should be evaluated and screened for metabolic syndrome. Prior to starting an SGA, providers should check baseline BMI, waist circumference, blood pressure, fasting glucose, and a fasting lipid panel. A personal/family history should also be established. BMI should be monitored at weeks 4, 8, 12, and then quarterly. If BMI is stable, it can then be followed annually. Blood pressure, lipids, and fasting glucose should be rechecked 12 weeks after an SGA is started. If patient is at goal, blood pressure and glucose can then be monitored annually, whereas lipids should be checked every 5 years. Waist circumference and history should also be monitored annually. **(p. 164)**

4. **The correct response is option B: They are unlikely to affect lithium levels.**

   ACE inhibitors and ARBs are first-line treatment in patients with high blood pressure and diabetes. Stage I hypertension is defined as average systolic blood pressure greater than 139 mmHg or average diastolic blood pressure greater than 89 mmHg occurring at two separate visits after an initial screening. It is important to note that use of an ACE inhibitor (as well as thiazides diuretics and ARBs) can increase lithium levels and increase risk for lithium toxicity. They can also cause hyperkalemia; therefore, a basic metabolic panel should be checked prior to initiating an ACE inhibitor, and rechecked shortly after starting or adjusting dosage. Patients should be informed that cough is the most common side effect of an ACE inhibitor, often requiring a substitution for the ACE inhibitor by an ARB, which has a low incidence of cough but similar benefits for blood pressure and kidney disease. **(pp. 169, 173–175)**

Clinical Case 2

1. **The correct response is option D: All of the above.**

   Switching to a medication with lower risk for obesity is a first-line intervention in patients who develop metabolic syndrome. In general, first-generation antipsychotics have fewer metabolic side effects than SGAs. Ideally, all patients with metabolic syndrome should be referred to a primary care physician (PCP) for intensive management. A nutritionist can help tailor diet to help treat the dyslipidemia, hyperglycemia, obesity, and hypertension. **(pp. 172–176)**

2. **The correct response is option D: Starting simvastatin 80 mg hs.**

   Each component of this patient's metabolic syndrome should be addressed and treated. Lisinopril is appropriate to initiate for better blood pressure control, whereas metformin can help control blood glucose levels and limit additional weight gain. Although Mrs. Heater does have dyslipidemia and should begin taking a statin, simvastatin 40 mg is a more appropriate starting dose. Higher dosages of statins are associated with more side effects, including myalgias and abdominal pain. If lipids are still not at goal after she has taken simvastatin 40 mg/day for 3 months, the patient should be switched to a more potent statin, such as rosuvastatin or atorvastatin. **(pp. 168, 172–173)**

3. **The correct response is option B: Discuss the importance of primary care and place another referral for a PCP.**

This patient's metabolic syndrome is still poorly controlled despite the interventions you have made, and will likely need more aggressive management. Therefore, Mrs. Heater needs to establish with a PCP as soon as possible. Absolute indications for referral to a PCP in this patient include blood glucose above 200 mg/dL despite treatment, and persistent blood pressure above 180/110 mmHg despite treatment. It is unlikely that a small dosage adjustment in her lisinopril will get her blood pressure to goal. Waist circumference should be checked annually in patients taking SGAs, not after just 1 month. A lipid panel should be checked 3 months after initiating therapy, not after 1 month. **(pp. 164, 174–175)**

4. **The correct response is option B: Refer for a sleep study.**

Mrs. Heater is doing much better, and her blood pressure and diabetes are now well controlled on her new medication regimen. She is tolerating the simvastatin, and her lipid panel is at goal. She is having symptoms of obstructive sleep apnea, which can be a common complication of obesity and the metabolic syndrome. A diagnostic sleep study is the best test to evaluate for this concern. **(pp. 172–174)**

CHAPTER 13

Osteoporosis

Clinical Case 1

1. **The correct response is option B: Osteopenia.**

   A T-score greater than −1.0 indicates normal bone density, a T-score between −1.0 and −2.5 indicates osteopenia, and a T-score below −2.5 indicates osteoporosis (Table 13–1). **(pp. 188–189)**

TABLE 13–1. World Health Organization diagnostic classification of osteoporosis

Category	T-score[a]	Bone mineral density
Normal	>−1.0	Within 1 SD of a young normal adult
Low bone mass (osteopenia)	−1.0 to −2.5	Between 1 and 2.5 SD below that of a young normal adult
Osteoporosis	<−2.5	>2.5 SD below that of a young normal adult
Severe osteoporosis	<−2.5 and ≥1 fragility fracture	>2.5 SD below that of a young normal adult

Note. SD = standard deviation.
[a]The T-score compares an individual's bone mineral density with the mean value for young healthy individuals and expresses the difference as a SD score.
Source. Adapted from World Health Organization: "WHO Scientific Group on the Assessment of Osteoporosis at Primary Health Care Level, Summary Meeting Report, Brussels, Belgium, 5–7 May, 2004." Geneva, Switzerland, World Health Organization, 2004. Available at: http://www.who.int/chp/topics/Osteoporosis.pdf.

2. **The correct response is option B: A comparison to bone mineral density of a healthy 30-year-old female reference.**

   A DEXA measures bone mineral density in the lumbar vertebrae (L1–L4) and the hip. The T-score is a comparison of the patient's bone mineral density to that of a healthy 30-year-old female reference and is used for osteoporosis diagnosis in postmenopausal women. A Z-score is a comparison to a reference matched for age, ethnicity, and sex; it is used for premenopausal women and for men younger than 50 years. The numerical value is the number of standard deviations above or below the comparison group. **(p. 188)**

3. **The correct response is option G: All of the above.**

   These are all risk factors for development of osteoporosis (Table 13–2). Patients with mental illness are at increased risk for osteoporosis. Contributing factors include psychotropic medications, lifestyle factors, comorbid alcohol and tobacco use, and mental illness itself. Other risk factors for osteoporosis include female sex, white or Asian race, age older than 50 years, weight less than 126 lbs, personal fracture history, first-degree relative with fracture history, medications (e.g., glucocorticoids, aromatase inhibitors, androgen deprivation therapy, psychotropic medications), and conditions associated with bone loss (e.g., hypogonadism, hyperthyroidism, hyperparathyroidism, Cushing's syndrome). **(pp. 184–185, 187)**

4. **The correct response is option C: Hyperprolactinemia.**

   Antipsychotics carry the risk of elevating prolactin levels, which in turn can have direct effect on bone resorption. Prolactin also is thought to inhibit secretion of sex hormones, which can affect bone homeostasis. Selective serotonin reuptake inhibitors and antiepileptics have also been shown to impact bone metabolism via different mechanisms. **(p. 185)**

Clinical Case 2

1. **The correct response is option A: Osteoporosis.**

   A presumptive diagnosis of osteoporosis can be made following a fragility fracture, regardless of the DEXA score. **(p. 188)**

TABLE 13–2. Risk factors for osteoporosis

Age >50
Female sex
White or Asian race
Prior fracture
First-degree relative with fracture
Current cigarette smoking
Excess alcohol use
Low body weight (<57 kg or 126 lb)
Medications: glucocorticoid use (e.g., prednisone 5 mg or equivalent for ≥3 months), aromatase inhibitors, androgen deprivation therapy
Conditions associated with bone loss: hyperthyroidism, hyperparathyroidism, hypogonadism, Cushing's syndrome
Psychiatric patients
Increased risk of fracture associated with psychotropic medications
Selective serotonin reuptake inhibitors
Antiepileptic drugs
Sedatives
Consider risk of hyperprolactinemia in patients taking antipsychotics
Consider risk of vitamin D deficiency in patients taking cytochrome P450–inducer antiepileptic drugs, elderly patients, and institutionalized patients

2. **The correct response is option E: Bisphosphonate and supplementation with calcium and vitamin D.**

   Pharmacological treatment of osteoporosis includes a bisphosphonate along with calcium and vitamin D supplementation. Lifestyle treatments, including tobacco cessation, alcohol reduction, weight-bearing exercise, and proper nutrition, are also indicated. Fall risk reduction is another important component of treatment. **(pp. 193–194)**

3. **The correct response is option C: Calcium 1,200 mg/day and vitamin D 800 IU/day.**

   For prevention of osteoporosis in *premenopausal* women and in men, calcium 1,000 mg/day and vitamin D 400–600 IU/day would be most appropriate. For prevention of osteoporosis in *postmenopausal* women and anyone with diagnosed osteoporosis, the current recommended supplementations are calcium 1,200 mg/day and vitamin D 800 IU/day. A vitamin D level below 30 ng/mL is insufficient and would warrant higher vitamin D repletion doses. **(pp. 191, 193)**

CHAPTER 14

Thyroid Disorders

Clinical Case 1

1. **The correct response is option C: Constipation.**

   Hypothyroidism is a functional thyroid disorder characterized by a constellation of symptoms (Table 14–1), including neuropsychiatric symptoms such as depressed mood, fatigue, poor concentration, and cognitive impairment; weight gain; cold intolerance; constipation; dry skin and coarse hair; ataxia; delayed tendon reflexes; irregular or heavy menses; bradycardia; and hypothermia. **(pp. 203–204)**

TABLE 14–1. Common signs and symptoms of thyroid dysfunction: hypothyroidism

Depression, fatigue, decreased concentration
Cognitive impairment
Weight gain
Cold intolerance
Constipation
Bradycardia
Hypothermia
Dry skin, coarse hair
Ataxia
Delayed deep tendon reflex
Irregular or heavy menses

2. **The correct response is option B: Start levothyroxine 25 µg/day, and measure serum TSH 6–8 weeks after initiating treatment.**

   Hypothyroidism is treated with levothyroxine. It is recommended to start levothyroxine 25–75 µg/day, based on degree of thyroid-stimulating hormone (TSH) elevation and comorbidities. A full replacement dosage of levothyroxine is generally about 1.6 µg/kg/day after thyroidectomy. For hypothyroid patients not requiring surgery, this dose may not be necessary, and the dose should be titrated over time given the likelihood of residual thyroid function early in the course of hypothyroidism. Serum TSH should be checked 6–8 weeks after levothyroxine is initiated, and again 6–8 weeks after any dose adjustment. Serum TSH monitoring can be decreased to every 3–6 months once a thyroid state is achieved. Additionally, any patient with a cardiac comorbidity should warrant caution by starting levothyroxine at a lower dose and titrating more slowly. **(p. 208)**

Clinical Case 2

1. **The correct response is option D: All of the above.**

   The American Academy of Clinical Endocrinologists (AACE), American Thyroid Association (ATA), and U.S. Preventive Services Task Force have varying recommendations regarding screening for thyroid disorders in the general population (Table 14–2). However, regarding patients with psychiatric conditions, the AACE and ATA agree that compelling evidence exists to support thyroid dysfunction screening, as described in the three options listed above. **(pp. 205–207)**

TABLE 14–2. Summary of screening guidelines for thyroid disorders

Obtain a baseline, screening serum TSH level as part of the initial workup of all psychiatric patients, particularly those who have affective and anxiety disorders.
Consider screening TSH in any patient over age 35 and every 5 years thereafter, particularly for women and elderly patients.
Screen elderly patients with any new or worsening cognitive dysfunction or mood symptoms.

Note. TSH = thyroid-stimulating hormone.

2. **The correct response is option C: Weight loss.**

   Apathetic hyperthyroidism presents with a paucity of symptoms that may suggest psychiatric disease. In elderly individuals, symptoms of thyroid disease may be mistaken for normal aging, cognitive changes suggestive of dementia, or mood disorder. Along with pregnant women, the elderly represent a population in which thyroid disease often presents atypically. **(pp. 202, 204–205)**

Clinical Case 3

1. **The correct response is option A: Lithium.**

   Lithium can cause hypothyroidism and goiter by decreasing the synthesis and release of thyroid hormone. Lithium also decreases activity of the enzyme that leads to peripheral conversion of thyroxine (T_4) to triiodothyronine (T_3). **(pp. 202–203, 209)**

2. **The correct response is option C: Erythrocyte sedimentation rate (ESR).**

   A significant percentage of patients (6%–52%) with antithyroid antibodies will eventually develop hypothyroidism while taking lithium, thereby warranting an antithyroid peroxidase antibody titer prior to lithium administration. In addition, TSH and free T_4 should be monitored regularly while taking lithium. There is no indication for checking an ESR. **(pp. 202–203)**

3. **The correct response is option B: Continue lithium and initiate levothyroxine 25 μg/day.**

   Lithium use increases the risk of hypothyroidism, which should be treated with levothyroxine. The development of hypothyroidism is not a contraindication for lithium use. **(pp. 202–203)**

CHAPTER 15

Adult Immunizations

Clinical Case 1

1. **The correct response is option E: Administer PCV13 today and have him return in 8 weeks for PPSV23.**

   This patient is particularly vulnerable to pneumococcal infection due to his chronic renal failure and therefore should receive both the PCV13 and the PPSV23, separated by 8 weeks to provide broader coverage against pneumococcal serotypes. **(p. 219)**

2. **The correct response is option B: Pneumococcal vaccine does not reduce the rate of pneumonia but does reduce the burden of bacteremia associated with pneumonia.**

   The pneumococcal vaccine does not decrease the rate of pneumonia but does reduce the burden of bacteremia and thereby lowers the mortality rate. Adults younger than 65 years may require pneumococcal vaccination if they have certain comorbidities, including chronic lung disease, cardiovascular disease, diabetes, chronic renal failure, nephrotic syndrome, chronic liver disease, alcoholism, cochlear implants, asplenia, cerebrospinal fluid leaks, or other immunocompromising conditions. HIV is an indication for pneumococcal vaccination. **(pp. 217, 219)**

3. **The correct response is option C: He should receive Tdap today and have a Td booster in 10 years.**

   This patient has gone over 10 years since his last tetanus booster. He should have a single Tdap (tetanus, diphtheria, and pertussis vaccine) to provide protection from pertussis. This vaccination with Tdap will be sufficient as a booster for tetanus, and his next Td (tetanus and diphtheria) booster should be in 10 years (Table 15–1). **(pp. 218, 220)**

TABLE 15–1. Overview of recommended adult immunization schedule

Human papillomavirus vaccine
All previously unvaccinated women up to age 26
Three doses on 0-, 2-, 6-month schedule
Do not give during pregnancy
Influenza vaccination
All adults in the fall or winter
Pneumococcal vaccine (Pneumovax)
All patients age 65 or older get once
Patients younger than age 65 with a chronic illness that predisposes them to pneumonia: chronic heart disease (e.g., congestive heart failure and coronary artery disease), chronic lung disease (e.g., chronic obstructive pulmonary disease, asthma), diabetes mellitus, chronic liver disease, chronic kidney disease, nephrotic syndrome, immunocompromise (due to disease or drugs)
Active smokers and those who chronically misuse alcohol
Patients living in high-risk settings (e.g., nursing homes, long-term care facilities)
For patients younger than age 65 who receive the vaccine, revaccination is recommended after 5 years or age 65, whichever comes first.
Tetanus-diphtheria (Td) or tetanus-diphtheria-pertussis (Tdap) vaccine
For adults who have had primary series, recommended to get booster of Td every 10 years
For adults younger than age 65 who have not had Tdap before, recommended to get once in place of Td booster
Varicella zoster vaccine (Zostavax)
All patients age 60 and older
Exclude patients with cellular or acquired immunodeficiency (e.g., those who have HIV or who are undergoing chemotherapy)

Clinical Case 2

1. **The correct response is option C: He should be vaccinated against hepatitis B only.**

   Persons with behavioral risk factors for hepatitis A include men who have sex with men, intravenous drug use, international travel, chronic liver disease, and occupational exposures. According to the history provided in the question, Mr. Spaulding does not have risk factors for hepatitis A. His diabetes is an indication for getting the hepatitis B vaccine. **(pp. 223–224)**

2. **The correct response is option B: He should receive the varicella zoster vaccine today.**

   The patient has no contraindications for varicella zoster vaccination and therefore should be vaccinated because he is 60 years old (see Table 15–1). There is no need to test for immunity to varicella prior to vaccination against zoster. **(pp. 218, 222–223)**

3. **The correct response is option D: All of the above.**

   Patients for whom varicella zoster vaccination is contraindicated include those with primary or acquired immunodeficiency from malignancy or HIV, those taking immunosuppressive medications (including high doses of glucocorticoids lasting 2 weeks or more), and those with evidence of impaired cellular immunity on laboratory testing. **(p. 223)**

Clinical Case 3

1. **The correct response is option A: He should be vaccinated against human papilloma virus (HPV).**

   HPV vaccine is indicated for men ages 22–26 years who have sex with men, because they are at increased risk of HPV infection and thus are at increased risk of acquiring conditions such as genital warts, anal cancer, and intraepithelial neoplasia. This vaccine is also recommended for all males ages 13–21 who have not been vaccinated previously. He does not have an indication for pneumococcal vaccination because he is younger than 65 years, and he received Tdap at age 18 so his next booster will be at age 28 with Td (see Table 15–1). **(pp. 218, 222)**

2. **The correct response is option C: Hepatitis B.**

   Medical risk factors for hepatitis B infection include diabetes, end-stage renal disease (including patients on hemodialysis), HIV, chronic liver disease, and any present or suspected sexually transmitted disease. Persons with behavioral risks include heterosexuals with multiple sex partners, injection drug users, men who have sex with men, and persons with household contacts or sex partners who have chronic hepatitis B infection. **(p. 223)**

3. **The correct response is option C: Varicella zoster.**

   Varicella zoster vaccine should not be administered to persons with primary or acquired immunodeficiency from malignancies, HIV/AIDS, or immunosuppressive medications (including high-dose steroids lasting 2 weeks or more), or to persons with evidence of impaired cellular immunity on laboratory testing. The remaining vaccines would be recommended for him. **(pp. 219, 221, 222, 223–224)**

CHAPTER 16

Sexually Transmitted Infections

Clinical Case 1

1. **The correct response is option B: Trichomoniasis.**

   The U.S. Preventive Services Task Force recommends annual screening for women with high-risk sexual behaviors for HIV, syphilis, gonorrhea, and chlamydia (Table 16–1). A common presentation of trichomoniasis includes vaginal discharge and urethritis, which the patient reports not having. **(pp. 231, 236)**

TABLE 16–1. Summary of U.S. Preventive Services Task Force guidelines on sexually transmitted infection screening

Sexually active women under age 25 should be screened annually for chlamydia and gonorrhea.
All women who engage in high-risk sexual behavior (multiple partners, new partners, inconsistent condom use, having sex under the influence of alcohol or drugs, having sex in exchange for money or drugs) should be routinely screened for chlamydia, gonorrhea, human immunodeficiency virus (HIV), and syphilis.
Pregnant women should be screened for syphilis, HIV, chlamydia, and hepatitis B at the first prenatal visit, as well as gonorrhea if at risk.
Men engaging in high-risk sexual behavior should be screened for syphilis and HIV.
There is no benefit to screening the general population for hepatitis B, herpes simplex virus, or human papillomavirus.

Source. Adapted from Meyers D, Wolff T, Gregory K, et al.: "USPSTF Recommendations for STI Screening." *American Family Physician* 77:819–824, 2008.

2. **The correct response is option D: Single 1-g dose of oral azithromycin and single 250-mg dose of intramuscular ceftriaxone.**

   Patients infected with gonorrhea are commonly coinfected with chlamydia. Therefore, it is recommended to treat both organisms (Table 16–2). Metronidazole is the treatment for trichomoniasis and is not indicated in this scenario. **(pp. 233, 236)**

3. **The correct response is option C: This case must be reported to public health authorities, and the patient should abstain from sex for at least 1 week.**

   New cases of chlamydia, gonorrhea, syphilis, viral hepatitis, and HIV must be reported to state public health agencies and the Centers for Disease Control and Prevention (CDC). The patient should abstain from sex for 1 week after treatment. Her partners should be treated. **(p. 236)**

Clinical Case 2

1. **The correct response is option C: Primary syphilis.**

   Primary syphilis typically occurs within 3–4 weeks after exposure to *Treponema pallidum* and results in a painless ulcer (chancre). Gonorrhea and chlamydia result in urethritis. Herpes simplex virus results in painful ulcers. **(p. 234)**

2. **The correct response is option C: Treat with benzathine penicillin 1.44 g intramuscularly once.**

   Treatment for primary syphilis is based on history and physical examination findings and includes a single dose of benzathine penicillin 1.44 g (see Table 16–2). Serological testing will not be positive for 6 weeks. In addition, the RPR and VDRL results will not change the need for treatment and are unnecessary. Acyclovir is the treatment for herpes simplex virus. **(pp. 233, 234, 239)**

3. **The correct response is option B: Refer this patient to an infectious disease specialist.**

   Penicillin allergy should be confirmed prior to choosing an alternative antibiotic treatment, because other treatments are less effective

TABLE 16–2. Summary of initial diagnostic tests and treatments for sexually transmitted infections (STIs)

Infection	Initial diagnostic test	Treatment: First-line	Treatment: Second-line (if available)
Chlamydia (*Chlamydia trachomatis*)	NAAT using 1) first-void urine or 2) urethral, vaginal, and rectal swabs	Azithromycin 1 g orally, single dose	Doxycycline 100 mg orally bid for 7 days
Gonorrhea (*Neisseria gonorrhoeae*)	NAAT using 1) first-void urine or 2) urethral, vaginal, and rectal swabs	Ceftriaxone 250 mg intramuscularly, single dose, plus either azithromycin 1 g orally, single dose, or doxycycline 100 mg orally bid for 7 days	
Trichomoniasis (*Trichomonas vaginalis*)	Culture, PCR, or antigen testing (depending on local availability) using self-collected vaginal or urethral samples	Metronidazole 2 g orally, single dose	Tinidazole 2 g orally, single dose
Syphilis (*Treponema pallidum*)	Dark-field microscopy or direct fluorescent antibody testing on exudate or tissue from the chancre; serology (VDRL) is useful 6 weeks after infection	Benzathine penicillin 2.4 million units (1.44 g) intramuscularly, single dose (see section "Treatment Recommendations" for details)	
Bacterial vaginosis (not exclusively an STI)	Gram staining and presence of clue cells in vaginal fluid	Metronidazole 500 mg bid orally for 7 days	
Herpes simplex virus	Viral PCR of ulcer swabs	Acyclovir 400 mg tid orally for 7–10 days	Valacyclovir or famciclovir

Note. NAAT = nucleic acid amplification testing; PCR = polymerase chain reaction; VDRL = Venereal Disease Research Laboratory.

at eradicating syphilis. This patient has a severe penicillin allergy and should not take the medication without specialist consultation. He should be referred to an infectious disease clinic for treatment options. Usually, skin testing will be done to confirm the penicillin allergy. The patient should abstain from any sexual contact until the condition is treated. **(p. 239)**

Clinical Case 3

1. **The correct response is option B: He should receive the meningococcal vaccine.**

   This patient lives in a dormitory setting and has never had the meningococcal vaccine. He had Tdap as a teenager, so his next dose would be 10 years from the date of Tdap vaccination with a Td booster. Hepatitis A vaccine is indicated for men who have sex with men and patients who request hepatitis A protection, travel to countries where hepatitis A is endemic, use illicit drugs, have laboratory or occupational exposure to hepatitis A, or have chronic liver disease or clotting disorders. Mr. Rush does not need the pneumococcal vaccine because he is younger than 65 years with no predisposing conditions. He could be considered for the human papillomavirus vaccine. He should abstain from sex until further assessment with his provider. **(pp. 220, 234)**

2. **The correct response is option C: Acyclovir 400 mg tid for 7 days.**

   The physical examination is consistent with herpes simplex virus infection, and preferred treatment is with acyclovir for 7–10 days. If Mr. Rush has frequent recurrences, he may require chronic suppressive therapy with acyclovir twice daily. Doxycycline and azithromycin are used to treat chlamydia, ceftriaxone is used for gonorrhea, and penicillin is used for syphilis (see Table 16–2). **(pp. 233, 239)**

CHAPTER 17

Viral Hepatitis

Clinical Case 1

1. **The correct response is option C: Screen asymptomatic or low-risk adults one time if they were born between 1945 and 1965.**

   According to the U.S. Preventive Services Task Force (USPSTF) and Centers for Disease Control and Prevention (CDC) recommendations, asymptomatic or low-risk individuals should be screened one time if born between 1945 and 1965 (Table 17–1). Additionally, all high-risk patients should be screened. High-risk factors include injection drug use, exposure via needle stick, reception of blood transfusion before 1992, and other chronic medical conditions such as long-term dialysis. **(pp. 250, 251)**

2. **The correct response is option C: Anti-HCV antibody.**

   Screening for hepatitis C virus (HCV) should be initiated with anti-HCV antibody; if positive, it can be followed up with HCV RNA and genotype. Although elevated serum transaminases are frequently seen in chronic HCV, levels can vary, and some patients can have normal levels despite active infection. In addition, serum transaminases are nonspecific findings of liver injury and are therefore not appropriate screening tests for HCV (Table 17–2). **(p. 249)**

TABLE 17–1. Screening recommendations for hepatitis B and C

Centers for Disease Control and Prevention	
Hepatitis B	Asymptomatic or low-risk patients—should not be screened
	High-risk patients[a]—should be screened
	Asian Americans and Pacific Islanders[b]—should be screened
Hepatitis C	Asymptomatic or low-risk patients—onetime screening for adults born between 1945 and 1965; otherwise, no screening indicated
	High-risk patients[c]—should be screened
U.S. Preventive Services Task Force	
Hepatitis B	Asymptomatic or low-risk patients—should not be screened
	High-risk patients[a]—no evidence for or against, no specific recommendations
Hepatitis C	Asymptomatic or low-risk patients—onetime screening for adults born between 1945 and 1965; otherwise, no screening indicated
	High-risk patients[c]—should be screened

[a]Sex partners of hepatitis B–infected persons, HIV patients, men who have sex with men, injection drug users, people born in countries with prevalence >2%, persons receiving immunosuppressive therapy.
[b]Anyone born in Asia (except Japan) or the Pacific Islands (except New Zealand and Australia); anyone born in the United States who was not vaccinated at birth and who has at least one parent born in East or Southeast Asia (except Japan) or the Pacific Islands (except New Zealand and Australia).
[c]Injection drug users, persons with recognizable exposure such as needle stick, persons who received blood transfusions before 1992, persons with medical conditions such as long-term dialysis.
Source. Adapted from Centers for Disease Control and Prevention: *Viral Hepatitis.* Atlanta, GA, Centers for Disease Control and Prevention, March 12, 2013. Available at: http://www.cdc.gov/hepatitis/; U.S. Preventive Services Task Force: *Screening for Hepatitis B Virus Infection: Recommendation Statement.* Rockville, MD, U.S. Preventive Services Task Force, February 2004a. Available at: http://www.uspreventiveservicestaskforce.org/3rduspstf/hepbscr/hepbrs.htm; U.S. Preventive Services Task Force: "Screening for Hepatitis C in Adults: Recommendation Statement." *American Family Physician* 70:1113–1116, 2004b.

3. **The correct response is option A: Hepatitis B (HBV).**

   There are inactivated vaccines available for HBV and hepatitis A virus (HAV). There is no vaccination for HCV, hepatitis D virus (HDV), or hepatitis E virus (HEV). The CDC recommends vaccination against HAV and HBV for high-risk groups, especially individuals with chronic liver disease (including chronic HCV), injection drug users, and men who have sex with men. **(pp. 250–251)**

TABLE 17–2. Diagnosis of acute and chronic hepatitis

Diagnosis of acute hepatitis	
Hepatitis A	+ IgM anti-HAV
Hepatitis B	+ HBsAg, + IgM anti-HBc, + HBV DNA ± HBeAg
Hepatitis C	+ Anti-HCV
Hepatitis D*	+ HDAg, + HDV RNA
Hepatitis E*	+ HEV PCR, + IgM anti-HEV
Diagnosis of chronic hepatitis	
Hepatitis B	+ HBsAg, + IgG anti-HBc, + HBV DNA ± HBeAg, IgM anti-HBc
Hepatitis C	+ Anti-HCV, + HCV RNA

Note. Anti-HAV = antibody to hepatitis A; Anti-HBc = antibody to hepatitis B core; anti-HCV = antibodies to HCV; anti-HEV = antibody to HEV; HBV = hepatitis B virus; HBeAg = hepatitis B e antigen; HBsAg = hepatitis surface antigen; HCV = hepatitis C virus; HDAg = Hepatitis D antigen; HDV = hepatitis D virus; HEV = hepatitis E virus; IgG = immunoglobulin G; IgM = immunoglobulin M; PCR = polymerase chain reaction.
*Not routinely tested in the United States.
Source. Adapted from Centers for Disease Control and Prevention: *Viral Hepatitis.* Atlanta, GA, Centers for Disease Control and Prevention, March 12, 2013. Available at: http://www.cdc.gov/hepatitis/Statistics/SurveillanceGuidelines.htm#GenCA.

4. **The correct response is option B: There is a cumulative 25% risk of interferon-induced depression.**

   A 2012 systematic review and meta-analysis of 26 observational studies showed a cumulative 25% risk of interferon-induced depression in the general HCV-positive population. Risk factors for interferon-induced depression include female gender, history of major depressive episode, history of psychiatric disorder, low educational level, and presence of subthreshold depressive symptoms at baseline. Psychiatric disorder is *not* an absolute contraindication to antiviral treatment for HCV. There is inadequate evidence to support prophylactic use of antidepressants as prophylaxis for interferon-induced depression. In unstable patients, psychiatric symptoms should be optimized prior to initiating treatment for HCV. **(pp. 253–255)**

Clinical Case 2

1. **The correct response is option B: –HBsAg, +IgG anti-HBc, +anti-HBs.**

   In the absence of HBsAg titer, positive anti-HBs and IgG anti-HBc indicate immunity from a natural HBV infection. Note that prior vaccination will lead to positive anti-HBs, but the anti-HBc will be negative. Hepatitis B is one of the hepatitis viruses with effective vaccinations. There is a high prevalence of chronic HBV in the Asian and Pacific Islander populations.[1] **(pp. 246, 249)**

2. **The correct response is option C: 75%–85% of HCV infections become chronic.**

   The majority of HCV infections (approximately 75%–85%) become chronic infections; the remaining 15%–25% of HCV infections are cleared. In contrast, an estimated 95% of individuals infected with HBV recover and do not develop chronic HBV. Fulminant hepatitis is a rare form of HBV. HDV can only duplicate in the presence of HBV. **(p. 246)**

3. **The correct response is option A: HAV and HEV.**

   HAV and HEV are acquired primarily via fecal-oral route. HBV, HCV, and HDV are acquired primarily parenterally, including via intravenous drug-use and unprotected sexual intercourse. HCV has a considerably low risk of sexual transmission; HCV can duplicate only in the presence of coexisting HBV infection. **(pp. 246–247)**

Clinical Case 3

1. **The correct response is option A: He is no more likely to experience higher rates of mania from interferon treatment than patients with no prior psychiatric diagnosis.**

   Several studies have supported that interferon-based HCV treatment can safely be delivered to individuals with psychiatric disorders. Cumulatively, there is no increased rate of experiencing symptoms from schizophrenia and mania compared with nonpsychiatric population controls. **(p. 253)**

---

[1]HBsAg=hepatitis B surface antigen; IgG anti-HBc=hepatitis B core antibody immunoglobulin G; Anti-HBs=hepatitis B surface antibody; IgM anti-HBc = hepatitis B core antibody immunoglobulin M.

CHAPTER 18

HIV/AIDS

Clinical Case 1

1. **The correct response is option C: Diagnosis of HIV infection early in the disease course.**

   Research has found that the earlier in the course of the infection that a patient is diagnosed, the better the outcome. Unfortunately, no HIV-targeted vaccine has been found to be solely effective. **(p. 260)**

2. **The correct response is option B: CD4 cell count.**

   After a positive HIV test is confirmed, the severity of HIV infection is largely determined by HIV viral load, CD4 count, and presence of opportunistic infections. **(p. 264)**

3. **The correct response is option B: History of receptive anal intercourse without barrier protection.**

   Receptive anal intercourse with no barrier protection is one of the top risk factors of HIV transmission identified by the Centers for Disease Control and Prevention. Other risk factors are listed in Table 18–1. **(p. 262)**

TABLE 18–1. Risk factors for transmission of HIV

Receptive anal intercourse without barrier protection with high-risk partner(s)
Receptive vaginal intercourse without barrier protection with high-risk partners(s)
Injection drug use
Noninjection illicit drug use (particularly stimulants)
Multiple sexual partners
Sex trade work
Exposure by health worker via hollow-bore needle-stick injury

Source. Adapted from Centers for Disease Control and Prevention: "Integrated Prevention Services for HIV Infection, Viral Hepatitis, Sexually Transmitted Diseases, and Tuberculosis for Persons Who Use Drugs Illicitly: Summary Guidance From CDC and the U.S. Department of Health and Human Services." *MMWR Recommendations and Reports* 61:1–40, 2012.

4. **The correct response is option D: Single-session sexually transmitted disease risk reduction interventions.**

   The most effective behavioral interventions supported by multiple clinical trials are single-session interventions. Effective interventions addressed education of patients on transmission of sexually transmitted diseases and skill building to improve likelihood of behavioral changes, such as condom use. **(p. 265)**

Clinical Case 2

1. **The correct response is option D: 180 cell/mm^3.**

   The pharmacological treatment for HIV infection is broken down into highly active antiretroviral treatment (HAART) and prophylactic medications to prevent opportunistic infections. Untreated HIV can cause the immune system to fail, and at certain CD4 counts, the patient becomes susceptible to infection(s). Prophylaxis for *Pneumocystis jirovecii* pneumonia is indicated for a CD4 count below 200 cells/mm^3. For a CD4 count below 50 cells/mm^3, prophylaxis against *Mycobacterium avium* complex is indicated. **(pp. 235, 266, 269)**

2. **The correct response is option B: Trimethoprim/sulfamethoxazole (TMP-SMX).**

   Under the guidance of an infectious disease specialist, patients with HIV infection whose CD4 count is below 200 cells/mm^3 require prophylactic medications for opportunistic infections. For a CD4 count below 200 cells/mm^3, prophylaxis against *Pneumocystis jirovecii* pneumonia is indicated with TMP-SMX. For a CD4 count below 100 cells/mm^3, prophylaxis against *Toxoplasma gondii* infection using TMP-SMX is indicated. Prophylaxis against disseminated *Mycobacterium avium* complex with azithromycin is indicated for a CD4 count below 50 cells/mm^3. **(p. 269)**

3. **The correct response is option B: Ritonavir.**

   Ritonavir increases the serum level of carbamazepine. A large number of antiviral medications for HIV infection interact with psychotropic medications (Table 18–2). It becomes especially important to review drug-drug interactions in patients on HAART. **(pp. 266–268)**

4. **The correct response is option A: Men who have sex with men.**

   Men who have sex with men (MSM), regardless of ethnic background, share the highest burden of disease. Half of individuals living with HIV infection in the United States are MSM. Notably, 45% of new diagnoses of HIV occur among young black MSM. About 16% of those living with HIV infection in the United States have a reported history of injection drug use. About 16% of new HIV diagnoses were in the Latino population, with women in the group having twice the rate of infection as men. **(pp. 260–261)**

Clinical Case 3

1. **The correct response is option D: Greater than three times the rate in the general population.**

   The prevalence rate for HIV infection among individuals with severe mental illness in both inpatient and outpatient settings was found to be 3.1%, over three times the rate in the general population. **(pp. 261–262)**

2. **The correct response is option B: HIV replicates slowly in its life cycle and develops resistance to antiviral medications if taken intermittently.**

   Because of the slow replication in the HIV life cycle, the virus has a high mutation rate. Resistance develops quickly to antiviral medications when taken alone or intermittently. Adherence to the first combination of HAART significantly influences the course of HIV infection. **(p. 266)**

TABLE 18–2. Important drug-drug interactions between psychiatric and HIV medications

Psychiatric medication class	HIV medication	Potential interaction
NNRTI	Efavirenz	*decreases* levels of bupropion
NNRTI	Nevirapine	*decreases* levels of fluoxetine and fluvoxamine
Protease inhibitor	Fosamprenavir	*decreases* levels of paroxetine
Protease inhibitor	Indinavir	*increases* levels of nortriptyline
Protease inhibitor	Lopinavir	*decreases* levels of lamotrigine
Protease inhibitor	Darunavir	*decreases* levels of paroxetine and sertraline
	Darunavir	*increases* levels of trazodone
Protease inhibitor	Nelfinavir	*increases* levels of desipramine
Protease inhibitor	Ritonavir	*increases* serum levels of carbamazepine, sertraline, citalopram, paroxetine, nortriptyline, desipramine, imipramine, amitriptyline, clomipramine, and doxepin
Protease inhibitor	Ritonavir	*decreases* levels of lamotrigine and olanzapine
Protease inhibitor	Tipranavir	*decreases* levels of bupropion
Azole antifungal	Fluconazole	*increases* levels of nortriptyline
SSRI	Fluoxetine	*increases* serum levels of amprenavir, delavirdine, efavirenz, indinavir, nelfinavir, ritonavir, and saquinavir
SSRI	Fluvoxamine	*increases* serum levels of amprenavir, delavirdine, efavirenz, indinavir, nelfinavir, ritonavir, and saquinavir
Phenylpiperazine antidepressant	Nefazodone	*increases* serum levels of efavirenz and indinavir

Note. NNRTI=nonnucleoside reverse transcriptase inhibitor; SSRI=selective serotonin reuptake inhibitor.
Source. Adapted from Repetto MJ, Petitto JM: "Psychopharmacology in HIV-Infected Patients." *Psychosomatic Medicine* 70(5):585–592, 2008; Watkins CC, Pieper AA, Treisman GJ: "Safety Considerations in Drug Treatment of Depression in HIV-Positive Patients: An Updated Review." *Drug Safety* 34(8):623–639, 2011.

CHAPTER 19

Breast Cancer

Clinical Case 1

1. **The correct response is option A: Nipple discharge that is bloody in character.**

   Classic symptoms of breast cancer include a new breast mass or lump that is hard, often painless, and mobile and that has irregular borders. Additionally, breast swelling, nipple retraction or discharge, and overlying skin changes such as erythema, thickening, or dimpling suggest malignancy. Some patients may have axillary lymphadenopathy that suggests spread of the disease to regional lymph nodes. **(p. 278)**

2. **The correct response is option B: Age and gender.**

   The two most important risk factors for breast cancer are gender and age; the median age at diagnosis is 61 years. Women are 100 times more likely than men to develop breast cancer. Other risk factors for breast cancer include a family history, particularly inherited genetic mutations like *BRCA1* and *BRCA2;* early menarche; late menopause; nulliparity or delay of childbirth past age 30; history of radiation to the chest wall; increased breast tissue density; history of proliferative breast tissue, particularly with atypia; use of exogenous estrogens; and race. The incidence in Asian Americans is lower than in Caucasian and African Americans. **(p. 276)**

3. **The correct response is option A: Referral for a screening mammogram starting at age 40.**

   Breast cancer screening guidelines vary according to which organization is publishing the guidelines. According to the American Cancer Society 2013 preventive guidelines, annual mammography is recommended beginning at age 40 and continuing for as long as the woman is in good health. A clinical breast examination by a health professional is recommended every 3 years starting at age 20 and annually for women age 40 or older. Breast self-examinations are an option for women in their 20s. Lastly, only women at high risk for breast cancer should undergo breast magnetic resonance imaging (MRI) in addition to annual mammograms. **(p. 280)**

Clinical Case 2

1. **The correct response is option A: Ultrasound-guided core needle biopsy.**

   Women who present with abnormal mammographic findings alone (i.e., have nonpalpable abnormalities) should undergo image-guided biopsy (Figure 19–1); this procedure is usually done with mammography, although ultrasound or MRI may also be used. Stereotactic core-needle biopsy is often performed on lesions only seen with mammography and is the standard approach for abnormal calcifications. Ultrasound-guided biopsies can be performed on lesions initially diagnosed with mammography that are also seen on ultrasound, as well as for palpable lesions. **(p. 279)**

2. **The correct response is option D: Breast hormone analysis.**

   Treatment is generally based on the risk of distant recurrence. This risk is determined by tumor size, lymph node involvement, tumor grade, hormone receptor status, and *HER2* status (Figure 19–2). For select patients, tumor gene assays may provide additional prognostic and predictive information. Depending on these factors, adjuvant therapy may be recommended. Breast hormone analysis is not a valid medical test. **(p. 282)**

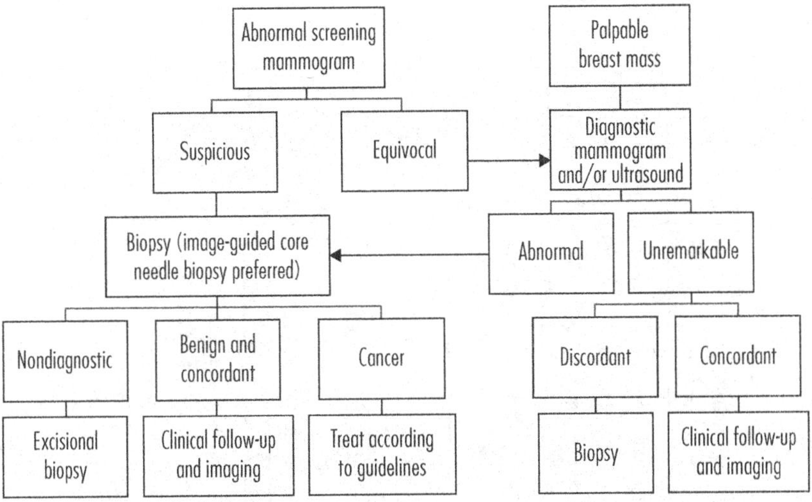

FIGURE 19–1. Breast cancer diagnosis.

3. **The correct response is option D: All of the above.**

Interactions between psychotropic medications and oncological therapies (e.g., chemotherapy, endocrine therapies, antiemetics) can result in adverse side effects. Certain antipsychotic medications, such as clozapine, can cause blood dyscrasias; when used in combination with cytotoxic therapy, these medications can lead to profound myelosuppression, causing life-threatening infections. Pharmacodynamic interactions between antiemetics and psychotropic medications, both of which independently prolong QTc, can lead to ventricular tachycardia. Therefore, close collaboration with the treating oncologist and psychiatrist is indispensable to good patient care. **(p. 285)**

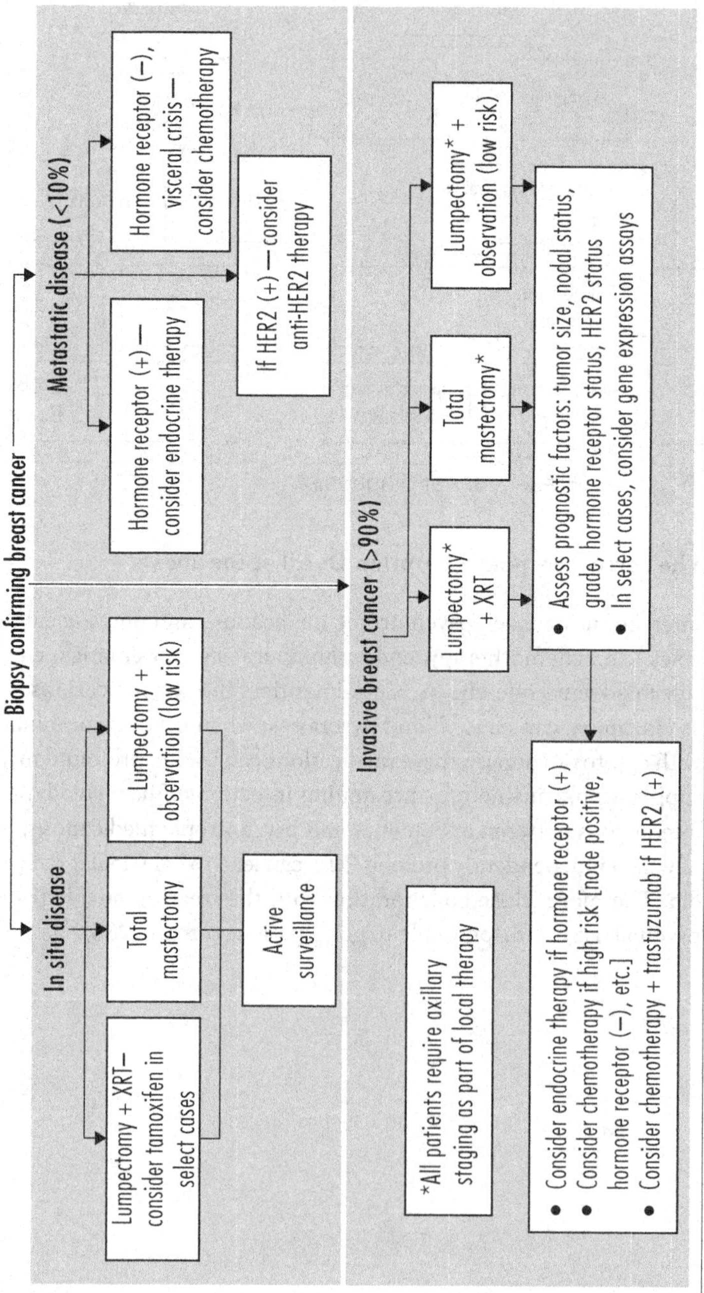

FIGURE 19–2. Breast cancer treatment algorithm.

Note. HER2=human epidermal receptor 2; XRT=radiation therapy.

CHAPTER 20

Prostate Cancer

Clinical Case 1

1. **The correct response is option C: Exposure to Agent Orange.**

   Risk factors for prostate cancer include African American ethnicity; family history; breast cancer susceptibility gene *BRCA1* or *BRCA2* mutation; Lynch syndrome; and, to a lesser extent, diet, insulin resistance, and obesity. There also appears to be an increased risk of prostate cancer in veterans with exposure to Agent Orange. A recent large retrospective study suggests that the incidence of prostate cancer is lower in patients with schizophrenia. **(p. 290)**

2. **The correct response is option A: PSA testing may lead to early detection of prostate cancer.**

   Prostate-specific antigen (PSA)–based screening for prostate cancer does lead to early detection of prostate cancer and likely reduces mortality, albeit to a small degree. However, the majority of prostate cancers detected by screening will not be fatal, or even symptomatic during the life of the patient. In fact, treatment of early prostate cancer can cause harm to the patient. It is generally not recommended to routinely offer PSA-based screening for average-risk individuals. **(pp. 292–293)**

3. **The correct response is option B: Referral to urology.**

   The traditional cutoff for an abnormal PSA test is 4 ng/mL. Any patient with an abnormal PSA test or digital rectal exam should be referred to a urologist for discussion of a transrectal ultrasound-guided biopsy that would help guide further treatment. **(p. 291)**

Clinical Case 2

1. **The correct response is option C: Anxiety.**

   Generally, psychiatric illness adversely affects the likelihood of screening. Patients with depression are less likely to be screened than nondepressed patients. Patients with anxiety are an exception in that they are more likely to be screened than nonanxious patients; the amount of screening for these patients is proportionate to the number of office visits. **(p. 292)**

2. **The correct response is option D: All the above.**

   The American Urological Association does not recommend screening patients who are younger than 40 years and older than 70 years. The American Cancer Society does not recommend screening for patients with a life expectancy of less than 10 years, as is likely the case for Mr. Godfrey because of his end-stage COPD. PSA-based screening is not recommended for average-risk individuals without symptoms, such as this patient. Patients with prostate cancer are also more vulnerable to developing psychiatric conditions, including posttraumatic stress disorder. **(pp. 290, 293–294)**

3. **The correct response is option C: Roughly 50% of men will have occult prostate cancer at the time of their death.**

   Prostate cancer is the second most common malignancy diagnosed in men after nonmelanoma skin cancer. Prostate cancer is a disease of age, and nearly 50% of men will have occult prostate cancer at the time of their death. Despite its high prevalence, the annual death rate from prostate cancer is very low, and men with prostate cancer confined to the organ at diagnosis can expect a survival rate of nearly 100% at 5 years. **(p. 289)**

CHAPTER 21

Lung Cancer

Clinical Case 1

1. **The correct response is option C: Smoking history.**

   There are many environmental risk factors in the development of lung cancer, including asbestos, pollution, and radiation. Male sex, older age, acquired lung disease, HIV, and family history can also place individuals at increased risk. However, the most important risk factor for lung cancer is cigarette smoking, which accounts for 90% of all lung cancers.

   Signs and symptoms of lung cancer are presented in Table 21–1. **(p. 300)**

2. **The correct response is option B: Computed tomography (CT) scan with contrast.**

   A patient with suspected lung cancer is usually first evaluated with a chest X ray. Suspicious lesions are usually followed up with a CT scan with contrast. The CT scan will better characterize a suspicious lesion, assess for enlarged lymph nodes, and determine extent of disease. After imaging, the next step is tissue diagnosis. This can be done via sputum cytology, thoracentesis, fine-needle biopsy, or CT-guided biopsy. After initial tissue diagnosis, further tests are often done to determine lung cancer stage (e.g., positron emission tomography [PET] scans, bone scans, and magnetic resonance imaging). **(p. 304)**

TABLE 21–1. Signs and symptoms of lung cancer

From primary tumor
- Cough
- Dyspnea
- Hemoptysis
- Chest pain

From intrathoracic spread
- Hoarseness (from recurrent laryngeal nerve palsy)
- Phrenic nerve paralysis
- Pancoast tumor (pain, skin temperature change, muscle wasting)
- Horner syndrome (ptosis, miosis, anhidrosis due to sympathetic nerve chain involvement)
- Chest pain (from chest wall or pleural invasion)
- Pleural effusion
- Superior vena cava obstruction (facial swelling, dilated veins on upper torso and arms, headaches)
- Pericardial effusion
- Dysphagia (from esophageal compression or invasion by tumor or lymphadenopathy)

From distant metastases
- Bone pain or fracture
- Lymphadenopathy
- Abnormal liver function tests, hepatomegaly, weakness (from liver metastases)
- Adrenal insufficiency (from adrenal lesions, rarely clinically evident)
- Headache, nausea, vomiting, focal neurological deficits (from brain lesions)
- Paralysis, bowel or bladder incontinence, sensory loss (from spinal cord compression by metastases)

From paraneoplastic syndromes
- Hypercalcemia (from parathyroid-related peptide or bony metastases)
- Hyponatremia (from syndrome of inappropriate antidiuretic hormone)
- Cushing syndrome (from ectopic adrenocorticotropic hormone secretion)
- Neurological syndromes (e.g., mononeuritis multiplex, encephalomyelitis, peripheral neuropathy, Lambert-Eaton myasthenic syndrome)

Source. Adapted from Beckles MA, Spiro SG, Colice GL, et al.: "Initial Evaluation of the Patient With Lung Cancer: Symptoms, Signs, Laboratory Tests, and Paraneoplastic Syndromes." *Chest* 123:97S–104S, 2003.

3. **The correct response is option D: Surgery, chemotherapy, and radiation therapy.**

Patients with stage II non–small cell lung cancer (NSCLC) would be treated with a regimen including surgery and chemotherapy, and possibly radiation therapy (Table 21–2). Stage I NSCLC is treated with surgery and possibly radiation therapy. Resectable stage III is treated with surgery, chemotherapy, and radiation therapy; and unresectable stage III is treated with chemotherapy and radiation therapy. Stage VI NSCLC is treated with chemotherapy or biologics or radiation therapy for palliation. **(p. 307)**

TABLE 21–2. Summary of treatment for lung cancer

Cancer stage	Treatment
Non–small cell lung cancer	
Stage I	Surgery ± RT
Stage II	Surgery + chemotherapy ± RT
Resectable stage III	Surgery + chemotherapy + RT
Unresectable stage III	Chemotherapy + RT
Stage IV	Chemotherapy or biologics or new targeted therapies
	RT for palliation
Small cell lung cancer	
Limited stage	Chemotherapy + thoracic RT
	Prophylactic TBI if response to therapy
Extended stage	Chemotherapy
	Prophylactic TBI if response to therapy

Note. RT = radiation therapy; TBI = total brain irradiation.

Clinical Case 2

1. **The correct response is option B: Smoking cessation.**

Primary prevention of lung cancer involves limiting exposures to known risk factors. The clinician's foremost goal in this case is to help the patient quit smoking. Secondary prevention includes screening for lung cancer and early identification. Blood pressure control has not been associated in primary prevention of lung cancer. **(pp. 302–303, 304–305)**

2. **The correct response is option D: All of the above.**

   The U.S. Preventive Services Task Force has made the following recommendations for lung cancer screening: annual low-dose CT (LDCT) screening for asymptomatic adults ages 55–80 years with a 30 pack-year smoking history and who currently smoke or who have quit within the past 15 years. Potential harms include a significant rate of false-positive LDCT results; 95% of all positive results do not lead to a cancer diagnosis. Many of these patients then undergo invasive procedures with their inherent risks and experience emotional stress from having a suspicious lesion. **(p. 305)**

3. **The correct response is option B: Limited-stage SCLC has a modest 5-year survival rate.**

   Limited-stage small cell lung cancer (SCLC) has a modest 5-year survival rate of approximately 20%–25%. SCLC accounts for approximately 14% of lung cancers, whereas NSCLC accounts for about 75%–80%. Extensive-stage SCLC is almost uniformly fatal by 5 years. Paraneoplastic syndromes are more commonly associated with SCLC. **(pp. 300–301)**

CHAPTER 22

Colorectal Cancer

Clinical Case 1

1. **The correct response is option A: Caucasian race.**

   A positive family history is one of the strongest risk factors for developing colorectal cancer. Other nonmodifiable risk factors include personal history of inflammatory bowel disease, diabetes, male gender, African American ethnicity, and increasing age. Common modifiable risk factors include obesity, smoking, alcohol consumption, and consumption of red meat (particularly meat cooked at high temperatures for long periods of time). **(pp. 314–315)**

2. **The correct response is option A: He presents with hematochezia.**

   Colorectal cancers are usually asymptomatic in the early stages. Screening tests are designed to screen a population before symptoms manifest. A diagnostic study should be pursued once an individual has the following symptoms: hematochezia, melena, changes in stool caliber, abdominal pain, weight loss, occult anemia, diarrhea, or constipation. Screening for colorectal cancer in average-risk individuals begins at age 50. Although patients with comorbid mental illness may need treatment optimization before screening, mental illness in itself is not a contraindication for colorectal cancer screening. **(pp. 315, 319, 323)**

3. **The correct response is option B: < 10%.**

   Most colon cancers evolve slowly from preexisting polyps over the course of 10–15 years. The most common type of polyp to evolve into a malignancy is an adenoma. The adenoma-carcinoma sequence is not well understood. Although all adenomatous polyps have malignant potential, less than 10% of adenomas will evolve to become adenocarcinomas. **(p. 314)**

Clinical Case 2

1. **The correct response is option B: Colonoscopy.**

   Fecal occult blood testing and fecal immunochemical testing can detect presence of blood in the stool, but both require colonoscopy for confirmation of positive results (Table 22–1). Flexible sigmoidoscopy examines only the distal colon, and a colonoscopy is necessary if abnormalities are detected. Computed tomographic colonography examines the whole colon but cannot remove polyps. Colonoscopy examines the whole colon, and polyps can be removed and biopsied. **(pp. 316–318)**

TABLE 22–1. Benefits and limitations of colorectal cancer screening methods

Test	Benefits	Limitations
Fecal occult blood test (FOBT)	Does not require bowel preparation Test completed at home Inexpensive Noninvasive Substantial research exists supporting improvements in cancer mortality	Requires multiple stool samples Poor detection of polyps Higher rate of false-positive results than other tests Pretest dietary limitations Colonoscopy necessary if abnormalities detected
Fecal immunochemical test	Does not require bowel preparation Test completed at home Noninvasive Fewer dietary restrictions than FOBT More specific for human blood than guaiac-based tests	Poor detection of polyps More expensive than traditional FOBT Colonoscopy necessary if abnormalities detected
Stool DNA test	Does not require bowel preparation Test completed at home Noninvasive Usually requires only one stool sample	Poor detection of polyps More costly than other stool tests Still being researched; adequate screening intervals uncertain Colonoscopy necessary if abnormalities detected

TABLE 22–1. Benefits and limitations of colorectal cancer screening methods *(continued)*

Test	Benefits	Limitations
Flexible sigmoidoscopy	Requires minimal bowel preparation Does not require sedation Substantial research exists supporting improvements in cancer mortality Lower risk of complications than colonoscopy	Examines only the distal colon Bowel preparation required May cause discomfort Cannot remove large polyps Small risk of bowel perforation Colonoscopy necessary if abnormalities detected
Colonoscopy	Examines entire colon Polyps can be removed and biopsied Can diagnose other colon pathology Required for abnormal results from all other tests Long interval between screenings	Full bowel cleansing required More expensive than stool testing Requires sedation Patients may have to miss a day of work Highest risk of complications compared with other methods No randomized trials illustrating mortality benefits
Double-contrast barium enema	Can view entire colon No sedation needed	Largely fallen out of favor as newer methods have developed Full bowel preparation needed Cannot remove polyps and often misses small polyps Exposes patients to radiation Colonoscopy necessary if abnormalities detected
Computed tomographic colonography	Noninvasively examines entire colon Performance is similar to optical colonoscopy for large polyps and invasive cancers Few complications No sedation needed	Full bowel preparation needed Cannot remove polyps Exposes patients to radiation Expensive May not be readily available in smaller centers or rural areas Colonoscopy necessary if abnormalities detected

Source. Adapted from American Cancer Society: *Colorectal Cancer Facts and Figures 2011–2013.* Atlanta, GA, American Cancer Society, 2011. Available at: http://www.cancer.org/acs/groups/content/@epidemiologysurveilance/documents/document/acspc-028312.pdf.

2. **The correct response is option B: Adjust the treatment for her panic disorder and reassess symptom control at her next visit before scheduling colorectal cancer screening.**

We recommend that colorectal cancer screening for average-risk individuals with co-occurring mental illness begin at age 50 (Table 22–2; Figure 22–1). The provider should begin by assessing the severity of current psychiatric symptoms based on the patient's level of impairment. Patients with well-controlled or mild symptoms should be screened with stool studies and sigmoidoscopy. For patients with moderate to severe symptoms, the clinician should first try to optimize treatment of the underlying psychiatric condition. **(pp. 320–321, 323–324)**

3. **The correct response is option D: A 44-year-old woman with schizoaffective disorder whose mother had colorectal cancer in her 80s.**

Patients should be referred for a diagnostic workup when they complain of symptoms or have signs of colorectal cancer. Additionally, asymptomatic patients with abnormal screening tests should be referred for further workup. Individuals with a history of a hereditary syndrome associated with colorectal cancer, radiation exposure, a personal history of colorectal cancer or inflammatory bowel disease, or a history of colon cancer in young relatives or multiple first-degree relatives should be referred for an individualized timeline for screening. **(p. 322)**

TABLE 22–2. Summary of colorectal screening guidelines for individuals

Organization	Initiating screening	Method of screening	Frequency of screening	Discontinuing screening
USPSTF[a]	All adults at age 50	Highly sensitive guaiac FOBT	Annually	Discontinue routine screening sometime between ages 76 and 85, although this decision should be made on an individual basis based on personal risks and health status; no screening beyond age 85
		Combined flexible sigmoidoscopy and highly sensitive guaiac FOBT	Sigmoidoscopy every 5 years, with FOBT every 3 years	
		Colonoscopy	Every 10 years	
		Computed tomographic colonoscopy	Insufficient evidence to support this as a tool for routine screening	
ACS-MSTF-ACR[b]	Average-risk adults at age 50	**Tests for early cancer detection**		Discontinue screening when life expectancy is less than 10 years
		Highly sensitive guaiac FOBT	Annually	
		Fecal immunochemical test	Annually	
		Stool DNA testing	Unknown	

TABLE 22–2. Summary of colorectal screening guidelines for individuals *(continued)*

Organization	Initiating screening	Method of screening	Frequency of screening	Discontinuing screening
ACS-MSTF-ACR[b] *(continued)*		**Tests for prevention and early cancer detection**		
		Flexible sigmoidoscopy	Every 5 years	
		Colonoscopy	Every 10 years	
		Computed tomographic colonoscopy	Every 5 years	
		Double-contrast barium enema	Every 5 years	

Note. ACS-MSTF-ACR = American Cancer Society, U.S. Multi-Society Task Force for Colorectal Cancer, and American College of Radiology; FOBT = fecal occult blood test; USPSTF = U.S. Preventive Services Task Force.

[a]Guidelines not meant to apply to patients with inflammatory bowel disease or specific hereditary syndromes such as familial adenomatous polyposis or Lynch syndrome.

[b]Guidelines designed for patients deemed to be at average risk for developing colorectal cancer.

Source. Adapted from guidelines provided by Levin B, Lieberman DA, McFarland B, et al.: "Screening and Surveillance for the Early Detection of Colorectal Cancer and Adenomatous Polyps, 2008: A Joint Guideline From the American Cancer Society, the U.S. Multi-Society Task Force on Colorectal Cancer, and the American College of Radiology." *CA: A Cancer Journal for Clinicians* 58:130–160, 2008; U.S. Preventive Services Task Force: "Screening for Colorectal Cancer: U.S. Preventive Services Task Force Recommendation Statement." *Annals of Internal Medicine* 149:627–637, 2008.

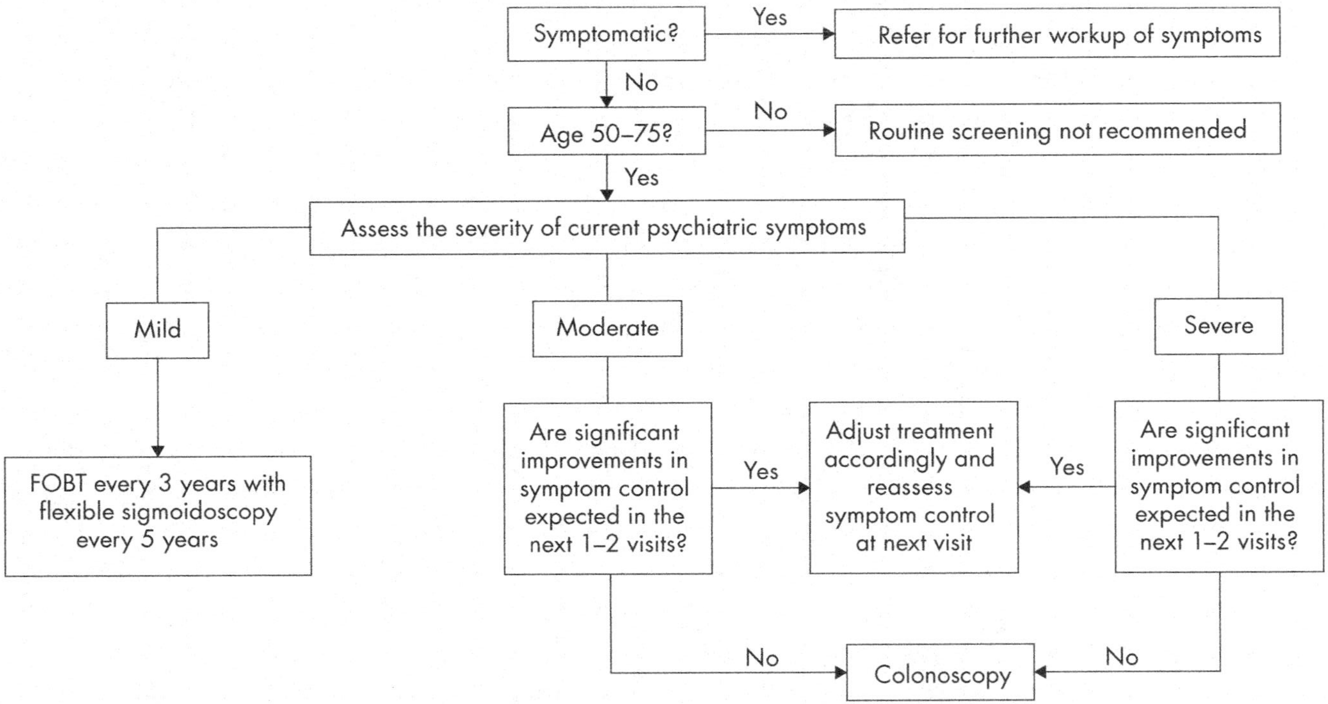

FIGURE 22–1. Colorectal cancer screening algorithm for average-risk individuals with comorbid mental illness.

Note. FOBT=fecal occult blood test.

CHAPTER 23

Cervical Cancer

Clinical Case 1

1. **The correct response is option A: Cytology every 3 years.**

   All guidelines recommend cytology (without human papilloma virus [HPV] testing) every 3 years between ages 21 and 29 (this patient is 23), and either cytology screening every 3 years or cytology and HPV co-testing every 5 years after age 30 (Figure 23–1). HPV vaccination does not affect screening recommendations. **(pp. 332–333)**

2. **The correct response is option E: All of the above.**

   You should inquire about why this patient feels uncomfortable with screening and then address those concerns directly. If she expresses misconceptions, providing accurate information and educating her is the most expedient action. Offering a personal recommendation for a primary care physician may lend credibility and help the patient feel more secure. Lastly, bringing screening visits into the mental health center can eliminate barriers to transportation and reduce anxiety of finding a new building (see Figure 23–1). **(p. 333)**

3. **The correct response is option C: Repeat cytology in 12 months.**

   For women with atypical squamous cells of undetermined significance (ASCUS) and negative HPV testing, the American Society for Colposcopy and Cervical Pathology (ASCCP) recommends repeat cytology at 12 months. Women with repeat ASCUS results or positive HPV serology should undergo colposcopy. **(p. 332)**

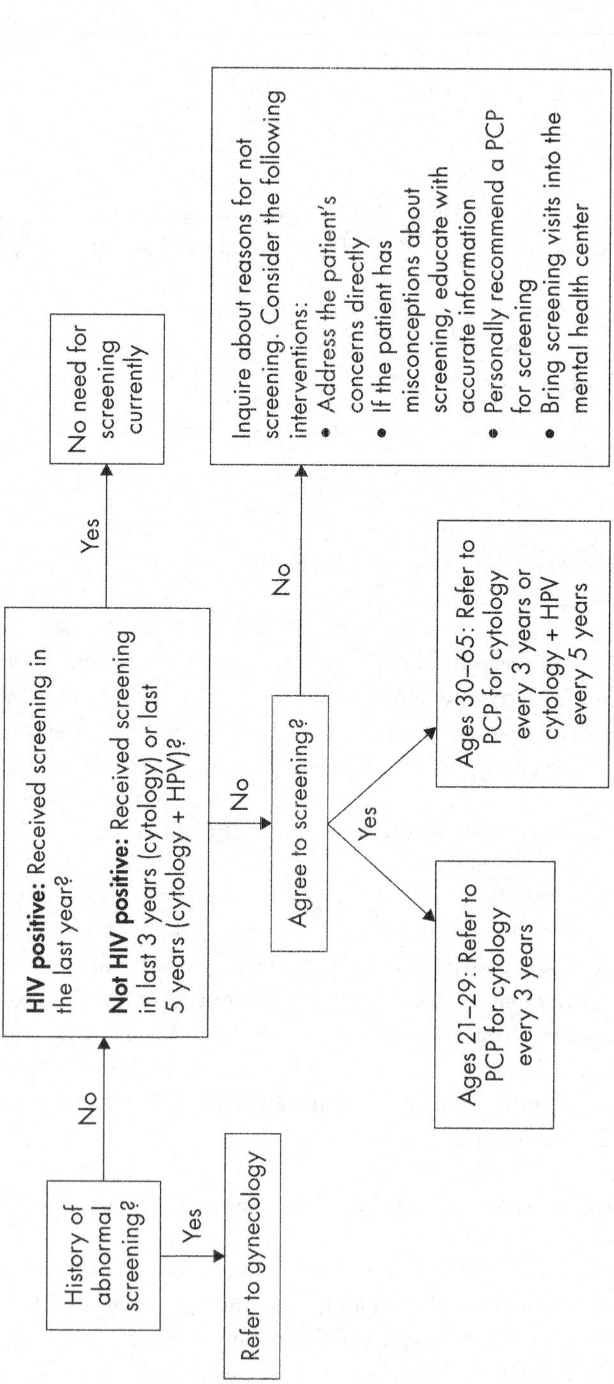

FIGURE 23–1. Screening for cervical cancer.

Note. HPV=human papillomavirus; PCP=primary care provider.

Clinical Case 2

1. **The correct response is option C: Peer education and support groups.**

   Methods to improve screening in those with mental illness include peer education and support groups. Mrs. Evans should also be screened for depression and anxiety disorders. Furthermore, decreasing out-of-pocket expenses, emphasizing early detection and treatment, and co-locating primary care and mental health care are all viable methods. An examination under anesthesia would not be appropriate for screening; however, if the patient has signs or symptoms of cervical cancer, referral to a gynecologist is warranted, where examination under anesthesia may be necessary. **(pp. 332, 334)**

2. **The correct response is option C: Cytology every 5 years with HPV cotesting.**

   All guidelines recommend either cytology screening every 3 years or cytology and HPV cotesting every 5 years after age 30. Because this patient is 35 years old, she qualifies for cytology and HPV cotesting every 5 years. **(p. 332)**

3. **The correct response is option C: Hysterectomy.**

   The ASCCP developed new guidelines in 2012 to guide the treatment of cervical intraepithelial neoplasia (CIN) lesions and adenoma in situ (AIS). Ablation and excision are both effective ways to treat CIN. Young women and pregnant women can be followed with serial colposcopy and cytology. AIS is ideally treated with hysterectomy for women who do not want to have children, but it can also be managed conservatively with excision and close follow-up for women who do want to maintain fertility. The latter option carries a risk of persistent AIS and progression to cervical cancer. **(p. 334)**

CHAPTER 24

Skin Cancers

Clinical Case 1

1. **The correct response is option D: All of the above.**

   Because exposure to UV light has been strongly linked to all types of skin cancer, sun protection is critical during childhood and beyond. This is most important in individuals with fair skin or a family or personal history of skin cancer. Additionally, exposure to tanning beds has been proven to increase risk as well as frequency of burns. **(p. 340)**

2. **The correct response is option A: Nodular basal cell carcinoma.**

   Nodular basal cell carcinoma appears mostly as a pearly, translucent papule with telangiectasias. It may also appear pigmented and can be mistaken for melanoma. Squamous cell carcinoma tends to appear as a firm, smooth, hyperkeratotic papule or plaque with a central ulceration. Actinic keratosis is classically described as scaly and erythematous macules or papules. Superficial spreading melanoma typically presents as an irregularly pigmented macule of plaque that is asymmetric with irregular borders of variegated color with a diameter greater than 6 mm. **(pp. 341–345)**

3. **The correct response is option C: It may result in significant tissue destruction and disfigurement if left untreated.**

   Basal cell carcinomas (BCCs) are typically slow growing, are sometimes associated with crusting and bleeding, and are primarily asymptomatic. Because they are slow growing, early detection and treatment is often successful. Metastasis is very rare. BCCs may result in significant tissue destruction and disfigurement if left untreated. The presence of actinic keratosis provides an opportunity for early detection and intervention to prevent progression to squamous cell carcinoma, not basal cell carcinoma. **(pp. 341–342)**

Clinical Case 2

1. **The correct response is option D: Superficial spreading melanoma.**

   Nodular basal cell carcinoma appears mostly as a pearly, translucent papule with telangiectasias. It may also appear pigmented and can be mistaken for melanoma. Squamous cell carcinoma tends to appear as a firm, smooth, hyperkeratotic papule or plaque with a central ulceration. Actinic keratosis is classically described as scaly and erythematous macules or papules. Superficial spreading melanoma typically presents as an irregularly pigmented macule of plaque that is asymmetric with irregular borders of variegated color and a diameter greater than 6 mm. **(pp. 341, 343–344)**

2. **The correct response is option B: Excisional biopsy.**

   Lesions suspected to be melanoma should be managed by excisional biopsy. Complete excision of a melanoma is important for two reasons: to provide a potentially curative effect and to determine the tumor thickness or depth of invasion. **(p. 345)**

3. **The correct response is option A: Severe mania or depression.**

   There are multiple new therapies under development for the treatment of metastatic melanoma. One of these treatments, interferon alfa-2b, has shown some success in treating patients with high-risk or metastatic melanoma. However, this treatment has also been found to be associated with adverse neuropsychiatric effects, including manic symptoms and severe depression. **(p. 345)**

CHAPTER 25

Geriatric Preventive Care

Clinical Case 1

1. **The correct response is option A: Iatrogenic fall.**

   Because Mr. Allen could not rise from his chair without using his upper arms, he has failed the Timed Up and Go test and thus likely had a recent fall due to use of antiarrhythmic and antidepressant medications. One in every three individuals over age 65 years suffers a fall, whereas the prevalence of elder abuse in the community is only 2%–10%. Both selective serotonin reuptake inhibitors (SSRIs) and antiarrhythmic medications are present on the 2012 American Geriatric Society Beers Criteria list and are modifiable risk factors for falls. Tricyclic antidepressants, SSRIs, anticonvulsants, antipsychotics, benzodiazepines, and nonbenzodiazepine hypnotics are to be avoided unless safer alternatives are not available. **(pp. 355, 357–359, 362, 365)**

2. **The correct response is option B: Reduction of diltiazem.**

   Reducing this patient's diltiazem can help decrease the risk for falls and address his bradycardia. Periodic reassessment of medication lists and deprescribing are recommended when possible to avoid polypharmacy for older adults. Rate control medications and anticoagulation, in the long run, are equal to or better than cardioversion. Compression stockings can be useful when postural hypotension contributes to falls. Reducing the patient's sertraline, which is included on the 2012 American Geriatric Society Beers Criteria, would not be the first-line treatment due to the patient's chronic elevated suicide risk (major depressive disorder and previous suicide attempt). **(pp. 355–364)**

3. **The correct response is option B: Secondary prevention.**

Mr. Allen already exhibits symptoms of falls—bruises, gait, and his failed Timed Get Up and Go test—and also has risk factors such as medications and a multiple-level house that may not be equipped with safety features. Primary prevention avoids disease and disability, whereas secondary prevention targets those (like Mr. Allen) who have risk factors or preclinical disease but who are otherwise asymptomatic. Tertiary prevention involves caring for those with established disease and preventing disease-related complications. Quaternary prevention reduces excessive screening and medical intervention and decreasing harm of medical care. **(pp. 16, 355)**

Clinical Case 2

1. **The correct response is option D: Cancer.**

Cancer is the most common cause of involuntary weight loss, accounting for 16%–36% of cases. Other causes include medical conditions, psychosocial issues, and medication side effects, can lead to involuntary weight loss (Table 25–1). SSRIs can lead to gastrointestinal upset. Depression, dementia, alcoholism, paranoia, and other psychiatric disorders can also lead to involuntary weight loss. Dysphagia, an inability to feed oneself, and an inability to obtain food can also cause weight loss. **(pp. 362, 364)**

TABLE 25–1. Common causes of involuntary weight loss in older adults

Medications (e.g., diuretics, serotonin reuptake inhibitors, benzodiazepines, β-blockers, metformin)
Psychiatric disorders (e.g., dementia, depression, alcoholism, anorexia nervosa, paranoia)
Difficulty with swallowing or chewing
Endocrinological disorders (e.g., hyperthyroidism, hypothyroidism, hypoparathyroidism)
Gastrointestinal problems (e.g., nausea, malabsorption)
Functional limitations (e.g., inability to feed oneself or obtain food)
Lower socioeconomic status (e.g., availability and amount of food consumed)

2. **The correct response is option A: A patient who is 75 years old with no history.**

   Screening for adults ages 50–75 is indicated, according to the U.S. Preventive Services Task Force (USPSTF) (Table 25–2). Routine screening is not recommended for adults ages 76–85, although there may be considerations that support colorectal cancer screening for an individual patient. Any kind of screening for colon cancer is not recommended for individuals ages 85 and older. **(p. 366)**

TABLE 25–2. Cancer screening guidelines for elderly patients

Cancer screening	U.S. Preventive Services Task Force (2013)[a]	American Geriatrics Society[b]
Breast	Screen using mammogram biennially women ages 50–74 years Insufficient benefit and harm of screening mammography in women age 75 years or older	Screen using mammogram annually or biennially until age 75 and at least every 3 years thereafter No upper age limit for women with estimated life expectancy of ≥4 years
Cervical	Screen with cytology for women ages 21–65 every 3 years, or combination of cytology and human papillomavirus every 5 years Recommend against screening in women older than age 65 years who have had adequate screening and are not otherwise at high risk for cervical cancer	Screen at 1- to 3-year intervals until at least age 60 Beyond age 70, there is little evidence for or against screening women who have been regularly screened in previous years
Colon	Screen using fecal occult blood testing, sigmoidoscopy, or colonoscopy for patients ages 50–75 years Recommend against routine screening for patients ages 76–85 but consider individualized assessment Recommend against screening for patients older than 85 years	No specific guidelines
Prostate	Recommend against screening	No specific guidelines

[a]U.S. Preventive Services Task Force: *Recommendation for Adults.* Rockville, MD, U.S. Preventive Services Task Force, 2013. Available at: http://www.uspreventiveservicestaskforce.org/adultrec.htm. Accessed May 25, 2013.

[b]American Geriatrics Society: "Breast Cancer Screening in Older Women." *American Journal of the Geriatrics Society* 48:842–844, 2000; American Geriatrics Society: "Screening for Cervical Cancer in Older Women." *Journal of the American Geriatrics Society* 49:655–657, 2001.

3. **The correct response is option C: Ask, "Have your belongings been taken from you without your permission?"**

   Screening questions such as this one can help assess elder maltreatment, which is a concern because this patient's caregiver has neither refilled the patient's medications nor taken the patient to his medical appointments. Elder abuse in this case is part of the differential diagnosis and should be assessed. However, screening for elder abuse remains controversial, because there is no standard screening tool, no universal guidance on whom to screen, and no standardized approach when abuse is identified. The USPSTF recommends against screening for someone of this patient's age (see Table 25–2). Refilling medications may be helpful, and mirtazapine can be used to increase appetite, but this would not be the next best step because this patient's appetite is already high. Screening for body dysmorphic disorder would not be helpful in this patient because he has no prior history of such a disorder. **(pp. 365–368)**

Clinical Case 3

1. **The correct response is option C: Inactivated intramuscular influenza and Tdap.**

   Ms. Scott will need Tdap because of a higher prevalence of pertussis infections in recent years (possibly due to attenuation of prior vaccinations) (Table 25–3). The Centers for Disease Control and Prevention recommends not delaying receipt of Tdap in patients over age 65, even if the most recent receipt of Td was within 5 years. Because it is autumn, the patient will also need an influenza vaccine. The live attenuated vaccine is available in an intranasal mist for nonpregnant patients ages 2–49 years old without high-risk medical conditions, and is therefore not recommended for the 66-year-old patient in this case. This patient can use either an intradermal or intramuscular inactivated influenza vaccine. **(pp. 218–220, 369)**

2. **The correct response is option D: Omega-3 fatty acid.**

   Regular fish consumption or omega-3 fatty acid supplemental intake is associated with decreased risk of all-cause dementia but does not prevent or treat those who already have dementia. The other listed sup-

TABLE 25–3. Recommended vaccinations for older adults

Vaccine	≥65 years old
Influenza	1 dose annually
Tetanus, diphtheria, pertussis (Td/Tdap)	Substitute one-time dose of Tdap for Td booster; then boost with Td every 10 years
Zoster	1 dose (starting at ≥60 years)
Pneumococcal polysaccharide 23	1 dose
Pneumococcal 13-valent conjugate	1 dose

Source. Adapted from Advisory Committee on Immunization Practices Adult Immunization Work Group; Bridges CB, Woods L, et al.: "Advisory Committee on Immunization Practices (ACIP) Recommended Immunization Schedule for Adults Aged 19 Years and Older—United States, 2013. *MMWR Surveillance Summary* 62(suppl):9–19, 2013.

plements have not been supported in large clinical trials to prevent or delay cognitive decline. **(p. 370)**

3. **The correct response is option A: Taking vitamins C and E.**

Ms. Scott suffers from age-related macular degeneration and scotomas (blind spots) with decreased fine visual acuity. Also, although unreported, the patient likely has loss of central vision. Cigarette smoking and low levels of antioxidants are risk factors. Vitamins C and E are antioxidants, along with zinc, which can help slow the progression of moderate and advanced cases of age-related macular degeneration. Because this patient is symptomatic, this can be considered tertiary prevention, not primary prevention. An ophthalmology referral may be indicated for assistance with management. **(pp. 355, 357, 361)**

Clinical Case 4

1. **The correct response is option A: Complete medication reconciliation.**

Although the other listed treatment options may be indicated in the future, the most important action at this time is a complete medication reconciliation. This process can facilitate the discontinuation of inappropriate medications to mitigate harmful side effects and drug-drug interactions. **(pp. 360, 362)**

2. **The correct response is option D: Inability to stand unassisted, walk 10 feet, and then return to seated position within 10 seconds.**

This option describes the Timed Get Up and Go test, which is a validated measurement in the prediction of falls in the elderly population (Table 25–4). The other answers have no clear relationship to fall risk. **(pp. 355–356, 359)**

TABLE 25–4. Gait components and office-based testing to indicate fall risk in older adults

Test	Abnormality in performance indicating fall risk
Gait observation	Hesitates, stumbles, or grabs or touches objects for support when initiating gait
	Weaves or sways side to side
	Scrapes or shuffles and does not clear floor consistently
	With turning, stops before initiating turn, staggers, has noncontinuous motion, or grabs objects for support
Timed Get Up and Go test	Is unable to rise from chair without use of upper arms, walk 10 feet, turn, and return to seated position in chair in <10 seconds
One-legged stance	Unable to maintain stance for 5 seconds

Source. Adapted from Tinetti ME, Ginter SF: "Identifying Mobility Dysfunction in Elderly Patients." *JAMA* 259:1190–1193, 1988.

3. **The correct response is option D: Orthostatic syncope.**

Lack of memory of falls as well as prodromal symptoms (lightheadedness and palpitations) suggests brief loss of consciousness, or syncope. Eliciting a detailed history from patients and caregivers is very important when assessing the etiology of falls. **(pp. 355–356)**

Clinical Case 5

1. **The correct response is option D: All of the above.**

At this point, it is important to consider a wide differential diagnosis when evaluating the patient's social withdrawal. Cognitive impairment, hearing loss (Table 25–5), and vision loss may all be contributors. **(pp. 359–360)**

TABLE 25–5. Screening questions and examinations for hearing loss

Questions	Examination
Do you feel you have hearing loss? Would you say you have any difficulty in hearing?	**Whisper test** While patient occludes one ear, examiner stands at arm's length behind patient and whispers 6 letter-number combinations. A positive test is failure to repeat half of the letter-number combinations correctly. **Finger rub** Examiner gently rubs fingers together at a distance of 6 inches from patient's ear. A positive test is failure to identify rub in >2 of 6 attempts.

2. **The correct response is option C: Open-angle glaucoma.**

   Open-angle glaucoma is characterized by painless loss of peripheral vision. Patients of African American race are at higher risk than those of other races. See Table 25–6 for characteristics of common causes of visual impairment in elderly patients. **(p. 361)**

3. **The correct response is option C: Zoster (shingles) vaccine.**

   Ms. Mason has multiple comorbidities and is dependent on caregivers for some of her activities of daily living. Her estimated life expectancy is 2–5 years. Thus, neither colonoscopy nor mammography is likely to be beneficial for her from a risk-benefit perspective. The herpes zoster vaccine is recommended for her age group. The meningococcal vaccine is recommended for adults who are traveling to endemic areas or who have medical risk factors (e.g., splenectomy, complement deficiency). **(pp. 220, 368)**

Clinical Case 6

1. **The correct response is option C: Given his excellent functional status, it is appropriate to send the patient for colonoscopy.**

   Although the USPSTF recommends against routine screening in patients ages 76–86, it suggests consideration of individualized assess-

TABLE 25–6. Four common causes of visual impairment in elderly patients

Diagnosis	Symptoms	Select risk factors	Preventive intervention
Age-related macular degeneration	Loss of central vision Scotoma (i.e., blind spot) Use of brighter light or magnifying glass for fine visual acuity Distortion of straight lines	Low levels of antioxidants Cigarette smoking	Zinc and antioxidants were beneficial in moderate and advanced cases in decreasing progression, but not for mild cases or primary prevention.[a]
Cataract	Loss of central vision Difficulty reading in dim light Glare with night driving	Cigarette smoking Excess sunlight exposure Corticosteroid therapy Diabetes	Limited prevention measures
Glaucoma	Loss of peripheral vision Painless unless closed-angle glaucoma	African American Increased intraocular pressure	Limited prevention measures
Diabetic retinopathy	Decreased visual acuity Floaters Curtain falling	Poorly controlled blood glucose	Glycemic, blood pressure, and lipid control; eye exam at time of type 2 diagnosis and within 5 years of type 1 diagnosis

[a]Evans JR: "Antioxidant Vitamin and Mineral Supplements for Slowing the Progression of Age-Related Macular Degeneration." *Cochrane Database of Systematic Review* 11:CD000254, 2012.

ment (see Table 25–2). Because this patient lives independently and has a life expectancy greater than 10 years, screening is reasonable. **(pp. 364–366)**

2. **The correct response is option A: Independent function, with or without chronic disease and with life expectancy of more than 5 years.**

   Mr. Moore is independent in his activities of daily living and instrumental activities of daily living. His chronic medical issues are well managed with medications, and he has no cognitive deficits and minimal physical disability. Primary prevention efforts are often most useful in this group of patients with greater life expectancy. **(p. 354)**

3. **The correct response is option D: Discontinuing omeprazole because of no evidence of active GERD.**

   Rational prescribing principles state that discontinuation of therapies when appropriate can be beneficial to patients (Table 25–7). Omeprazole can be discontinued because the patient is no longer experiencing GERD symptoms. Simvastatin would be recommended in this patient for cardiovascular risk reduction and should not be discontinued. Screening for cognitive impairment in this independent patient who continues to perform well in a demanding job is unlikely to yield useful information. Screening for prostate cancer with PSA is not recommended (see Table 25–2). **(pp. 360–363)**

Clinical Case 7

1. **The correct response is option B: Kindly ask the patient's daughter to step out of the room, and then ask the patient, "Do you feel uncomfortable with anyone who is taking care of you?"**

   Any concern for elder abuse should prompt further inquiry (Table 25–8). The question listed above is an appropriate question at this time. If you are unable to elicit further information, it may be appropriate to contact adult protective services. Failure of a health care provider to report suspected elder abuse is a criminal act—not to mention potentially dangerous for the patient. **(pp. 365, 367–368)**

TABLE 25–7. Rational drug prescribing for older adults

Practical steps to consider in optimizing prescribing to older adults	Comment
Request patients to "brown bag" their medications and bring them to clinical visits.	Ask patients to bring in all their prescription and over-the-counter medicines, supplements, and herbal drugs being taken to accurately reconcile medications.
When starting a new drug, set a 1) therapeutic goal and 2) therapeutic time frame.	Establish a therapeutic goal and time frame to reassess clinically the efficacy for each medication and reduce polypharmacy.
Start low and go slow.	Start medications at low doses and titrate up to the lowest effective dose to limit untoward effects of drugs.
Avoid prescription cascades.	Evaluate whether medications may be causing side effects that are misdiagnosed as symptoms, triggering prescription of additional medication to treat the drug's side effect.
Look for drug-drug and drug-disease interactions, and potentially inappropriate medications.	Refer to the Beers Criteria[a] and other pharmacology texts.
Limit medication changes to one or two per clinical encounter.	Avoid too many medication changes at a single visit because of potential miscommunication and/or adverse drug events.
Deprescribe when possible.[b]	Periodically reassess: ask for patient and/or family preferences, look for clinical indications, review for potential harm, and assess medication utilization.

[a]American Geriatrics Society: "American Geriatrics Society Updated Beers Criteria for Potentially Inappropriate Medication Use in Older Adults." *Journal of the American Geriatrics Society* 60:616–631, 2012.
[b]Bain KT, Holmes HM, Beers MH, et al.: "Discontinuing Medication: A Novel Approach for Revising the Prescribing Stage of the Medication-Use Process." *Journal of the American Geriatrics Society* 56:1946–1952, 2008.

TABLE 25–8. Screening questions for elder maltreatment

Who makes up your social support?
Who makes decisions about your life, such as how you should live or where you should live?
Do you feel uncomfortable with anyone who is taking care of you?
Has anyone forced you to do things you did not want to do?
Has anyone prevented you from getting food, medications, or medical care, or from being with people whom you want to be with?
Have your belongings been taken from you without your permission?
Has anyone close to you hurt you or harmed you recently?
Has someone talked with you who made you feel ashamed or threatened?

2. **The correct response is option B: 2%–10%.**

   Elder abuse, also called *elder maltreatment,* is an entity that describes physical, emotional, sexual, or financial abuse of older adults, as well as neglect. Studies of community-dwelling adults have reported prevalence rates of 2%–10%. **(p. 365)**

3. **The correct response is option A: Depression and cognitive impairment.**

   Dementia, cognitive impairment, and psychiatric illnesses such as depression are risk factors for elder abuse. None of the other listed options have been shown to be risk factors for elder mistreatment. **(p. 368)**

Clinical Case 8

1. **The correct response is option D: Answers A and C.**

   In evaluating weight loss in the elderly, it is important to consider a broad differential. It is imperative to conduct a thorough medication reconciliation to evaluate for polypharmacy, as well as a review of systems to evaluate other possible causes of weight loss prior to ordering diagnostic tests. **(pp. 362, 364)**

2. **The correct response is option C: Hyperthyroidism.**

   The symptoms of palpitations, gastrointestinal disturbance, and rapid weight loss in conjunction with the patient's chief complaint of worsening anxiety are all concerning for hyperthyroidism. Metoprolol, sertraline, and malignancy are also known causes of weight loss in elderly patients (see Table 25–1 earlier in this chapter). Anorexia of old age may occur in patients with poor functional status and multiple medical comorbidities, which is true of this patient; however, weight loss associated with anorexia of old age is usually not as rapid and is not typically associated with increased anxiety and gastrointestinal disturbance. **(pp. 202–203, 206, 362, 364, 394)**

3. **The correct response is option D: Colonoscopy and mammography.**

   According to USPSTF recommendations (see Table 25–2), colon cancer screening is indicated for individuals ages 50–75, and breast cancer screening is indicated for women ages 50–74. Cervical cancer screening is not recommended after age 65 in women who have had adequate screening and are not otherwise at high risk for cervical cancer. **(pp. 364–368)**

Clinical Case 9

1. **The correct response is option A: Thyroid-stimulating hormone (TSH) test.**

   TSH testing is indicated to screen for hyperthyroidism or hypothyroidism in elderly patients who present with worsening cognitive function or worsening mood symptoms. The other tests may relate to risk factors for vascular dementia but are of little use in the workup of worsening cognitive function in this patient. **(pp. 206–207)**

2. **The correct response is option A: Recommend that the daughter-in-law stop giving lorazepam to the patient.**

   Recognizing potentially inappropriate medications is important in rational prescribing. According to the 2012 American Geriatric Association Beers Criteria, it is advised to avoid benzodiazepines such as lorazepam for in older adults because of adverse drug events. Polypharmacy is the most likely cause of increased agitation in the setting of a new medication (lorazepam) that was not prescribed by a physician. It is important to educate patients and caregivers on appropriate use of medication. **(pp. 360, 362)**

3. **The correct response is option B: Recommend that the patient obtain an influenza vaccine.**

   This patient, age 79, is due for the influenza vaccination during the current flu season. He will not need another Td boost until 10 years after his last dose. He does not require any more doses of pneumococcal vaccine because he received his last dose after age 65 (see Table 25–3). According to the 2013 USPSTF recommendations, patients should be screened for colon cancer between ages 50 and 75 years but only on a case-by-case basis after age 75. Because this patient did not endorse symptoms consistent with a possible gastrointestinal bleed, there is no indication for colonoscopy. Omega-3 fatty acids may help with prevention of cognitive decline, but research has not shown it to be beneficial at slowing cognitive decline in individuals who already have dementia. **(pp. 366, 368–370)**

Clinical Case 10

1. **The correct response is option D: All of the above.**

   In assessing falls in the elderly, the clinician needs to obtain a thorough history that includes associated symptoms, fall location, and activities at the time of fall, as well as consider modifiable risk factors (Table 25–9). Basic neurological screening for neuropathy and assessments of visual or hearing changes are also important. Vitamin D insufficiency testing can also be considered. Given that Mr. Zima is undergoing palliative chemotherapy and radiation, he is at risk for multiple causes of falls, including postural hypotension, muscle weakness, sensory changes including peripheral neuropathy, and malnutrition in the setting of recurrent vomiting. **(pp. 355–358)**

2. **The correct response is option B: Discuss with the patient the likely diagnosis of cardiac arrhythmia and the risks and benefits of treatment versus no treatment.**

   This patient likely has a cardiac arrhythmia, which causes his recurrent falls. Given that his life expectancy is less than 2 years, he would need to understand the risks and benefits associated with any intervention (medication vs. procedures) for his diagnosis. Focus should be on quality of life, and discussion with the patient would be necessary to ascertain his wishes with regard to treatment. **(p. 367)**

TABLE 25–9. Modifiable risk factors for falls in community-dwelling older adults

Risk factor	Intervention
Movement and balance	
Gait abnormality	Group exercise
Muscle weakness	Individualized exercise program
Poor balance	Tai chi
Vitamin D insufficiency	Vitamin D supplementation: ≥800 international units daily, unless deficient
Environmental hazards	Home safety assessment and modification
Cardiac arrhythmia	Cardiac pacemaker or implantable cardioverter defibrillator
Diminished visual acuity	
Cataracts	Cataract removal surgery
Use of multifocal glasses	Single-lens glasses
Medication	
Class of medication	Reduction in and/or gradual withdrawal of medications, including psychotropics, diuretics, antihypertensives, antiarrhythmics, anticonvulsants, and anticholinergics
Number of medications	Four or more medications increase falls
Podiatric conditions	
Foot pain	Podiatry referral
Poor footwear	Discourage walking in high heels, bare feet, or socks indoors; an ideal shoe has a low heel, a supported heel collar, and a thin, firm, and slip-resistant sole
Postural hypotension	Reduce offending medication(s) that is affecting blood pressure
	Use compression stockings
	Slowly rise, in stages, from supine to seated to standing; perform isometric handgrips when standing; and increase fluid and/or salt intake

Source. Adapted from Gillespie LD, Robertson MC, Gillespie WJ, et al.: "Interventions for preventing falls in older people living in the community." *Cochrane Database System Review* 9:CD007146, 2012.

3. **The correct response is option D: Consider discussion regarding discontinuing simvastatin.**

   Mr. Zima has a life expectancy of less than 2 years and is nearing the end of life. Given his short life expectancy, vision and hearing screening have a lower priority. The focus should be on his quality of life, and it is not advised to perform cancer screening in older adults with a life expectancy of less than 2 years. Reviewing the medication list and discussing options for possible discontinuation of medication will help focus treatment options toward improving the patient's quality of life. **(pp. 364–365)**

Clinical Case 11

1. **The correct response is option B: Order DEXA and use the lowest two T-scores.**

   USPSTF 2011 guidelines recommend screening using DEXA for all women over age 65 years. DEXA composite scores can be normal, so the lowest two T-scores are recommended to guide therapy. The density of an individual vertebra can be decreased to the osteoporotic range while arthritic changes can increase the bone mass of other vertebra, causing the other T-scores to be higher. Although some evidence exists that computed tomography scans can be used to gauge bone mineral density, there are not yet any validated measures for their use. **(pp. 188, 190–191; see also Chapter 13, "Osteoporosis")**

2. **The correct response is option C: Answers A and B.**

   The SSRI escitalopram has been approved by the U.S. Food and Drug Administration (FDA) for major depressive disorder, and the atypical antipsychotic aripiprazole has FDA approval as an adjunct for major depressive disorder. Both of these medications may have an impact on bone metabolism. Antipsychotics may cause hyperprolactinemia, increasing bone resorption and inhibition of sex hormones, which are important for bone homeostasis. The mechanism of action of SSRIs remains unknown; however, serotonin receptors are found on osteoclasts and osteoblasts, suggesting that serotonin may have an important regulatory role in bone metabolism. **(p. 186)**

3. **The correct response is option A: Ask questions from the Cultural Formulation Interview, including "What troubles you most about your problem?"**

   The DSM-5 Cultural Formulation Interview can help increase patient-doctor understanding, especially in the context of a patient's cultural background. In this case, Ms. Quan reveals a significant trauma history in the context of the culturally informed interview. Her missed appointments, previous history of flashbacks, and previous suicide attempts may reveal undiagnosed posttraumatic stress disorder. The patient reveals that she emigrated from Indonesia in 1998, when riots, gang rape of Chinese women, and persecution of Chinese inhabitants occurred in that country. Increased understanding and cultural sensitivity can improve patient engagement in treatment. **(pp. 26–27, 194)**

Clinical Case 12

1. **The correct response is option C: Encourage her to consider increasing exercise and vegetables in her diet because evidence suggests that these measures may be helpful in slowing cognitive decline.**

   Research has shown that increased physical activity is associated with modestly improved cognitive scores. Increased consumption of vegetables is associated with a lower risk of dementia and slowed cognitive decline. Ginkgo biloba and omega-3 fatty acids have not been proven to slow cognitive decline in patients with current cognitive impairment. **(pp. 369–370)**

2. **The correct response is option C: Inform the patient that the next best option would be to undergo cognitive training to improve current cognitive functioning.**

   Cognitive training, particularly training that focuses on cognitive exercises rather than memory strategies, has been clinically proven to improve memory-related outcomes. Folic acid, vitamin B_6, vitamin B_{12}, and antioxidants such as vitamins E and C have not been found to improve cognitive function. **(p. 370)**

3. **The correct response is option C: Tertiary prevention.**

   Tertiary prevention would be the most appropriate label because the patient already has mild cognitive impairment. The goal of tertiary prevention is to slow the progression of the already clinically apparent disease or illness. Primary prevention aims to avoid disease and disability, and secondary prevention attempts to target and to treat asymptomatic older adults who have risk factors or preclinical disease. **(p. 355)**

CHAPTER 26

Child and Adolescent Preventive Care

Clinical Case 1

1. **The correct response is option E: All of the above.**

   Various studies have reported that prenatal exposure to tobacco or lead, as well as psychosocial adversity, may increase a child's risk of developing attention-deficit/hyperactivity disorder (ADHD). **(p. 378)**

2. **The correct response is option C: Twin studies suggest that heritability of ADHD is very strong.**

   The genetic architecture of ADHD is complex. Despite the identification of multiple candidate genes, studies have not identified gene variants at a statistically significant level. There is likely a strong genetic component to the disorder. Twin studies suggest that heritability of ADHD may be as high as 76%. **(p. 378)**

3. **The correct response is option D: 7%–9%.**

   ADHD is one of the most common psychiatric disorders in children and adolescents. Approximately 9% of individuals ages 13–18 in the United States are affected by ADHD. Symptoms are characterized by hyperactivity, impulsivity, and poor sustained attention. **(p. 378)**

Clinical Case 2

1. **The correct response is option A: Maternal exposure to the antiepileptic drug valproate.**

   Risk factors for autism spectrum disorder (ASD) include maternal and paternal age, low birth weight, gestational age, newborn hypoxia, and maternal exposure to valproate. Despite significant attention in the lay literature, no relationship has been found between specific foods or vaccines and risk of ASD. **(p. 379)**

2. **The correct response is option B: Daily maternal prenatal vitamins.**

   Unsurprisingly, both environment and genetics contribute to risk for developing ASD. Prenatal care throughout the entire pregnancy is important for many reasons. For example, regular visits may identify risk factors for low birth weight babies (one risk factor in the development of ASD). There is no screening test for ASD. Prenatal vitamins may decrease the risk of ASD. **(p. 379)**

3. **The correct response is option B: 400 μg/day.**

   For all women of reproductive age, 400 μg, or 0.4 mg, per day of folic acid is recommended. Children of mothers receiving folic acid supplementation had half the incidence of ASD as those whose mothers did not receive folic acid supplementation. Women who have a history of giving birth to a child with a neural tube defect should be instructed to supplement with 4.0 mg/day. **(p. 379)**

Clinical Case 3

1. **The correct response is option A: Cognitive-behavioral therapy (CBT).**

   Considerable evidence supports CBT with a specific trauma component for the treatment of posttraumatic stress disorder (PTSD) in children and adolescents. Psychotropic medications should be used sparingly and only in severe treatment-refractory situations. Dyadic caregiver-child interventions are appropriate for very young children with PTSD. **(p. 380)**

2. **The correct response is option C: In pediatric studies, propranolol has not been observed to be effective in PTSD prevention.**

   Few medications have been investigated to prevent PTSD in children. Propranolol has demonstrated efficacy in double-blind controlled trials for secondary prevention in PTSD in adults. This medication may modify the stress response system (sympathetic nervous system). However, propranolol has not demonstrated effectiveness in PTSD prevention in pediatric populations. **(p. 380)**

3. **The correct response is option B: Substance use disorder.**

   PTSD in youths is associated with significant psychiatric comorbidity, including depressive and substance use disorders as well as suicide attempts. Essential hypertension, weight gain, and arrhythmias have not been associated with PTSD. **(pp. 379–380)**

Clinical Case 4

1. **The correct response is option B: Body mass index (BMI) percentile.**

   Mental health providers should monitor the BMI of all patients, regardless of whether they are taking medications that have the potential for metabolic side effects. The mental health provider should coordinate treatment for obesity with the patient's primary care provider. **(p. 381)**

2. **The correct response is option A: Fasting blood sugar or glycosylated hemoglobin (HbA_{1c}).**

   Before a pediatric patient begins taking a second-generation antipsychotic (SGA) and at regular intervals, the clinician should obtain waist circumference, weight, BMI, blood pressure, and a lipid profile. The patient should also be evaluated for glucose dysregulation using either a fasting blood glucose level or the HbA_{1c} (Table 26–1). The patient's personal and family medical history should also be reviewed. **(pp. 381–382)**

3. **The correct response is option D: At each visit.**

   Once a child or adolescent has started taking an SGA, he or she should receive close metabolic monitoring (see Table 26–1). Waist circumfer-

TABLE 26–1. Metabolic monitoring in pediatric patients treated with second-generation antipsychotics

	Baseline	Each visit	3 months	6 months	Annually
Personal and family medical history	X				X
HbA_{1c}, fasting blood glucose	X		X[a]		
Waist circumference	X	X			
Weight[b]	X	X			
BMI	X	X			
Blood pressure	X		X[a]		
Lipid profile	X		X[a]		

Note. BMI = body mass index; HbA_{1c} = hemoglobin A_{1c}.
[a]After 3 months, follow-up every 6 months.
[b]Percentile.
Source. Adapted from Correll CU: "Monitoring and Management of Antipsychotic-Related Metabolic and Endocrine Adverse Events in Pediatric Patients." *International Review of Psychiatry* 20:195–201, 2008.

ence, weight, and BMI should be recorded at each visit. In addition, blood pressure, lipid profile, and either a fasting blood glucose or HbA_{1c} should be measured 3 months after starting the SGA and every 6 months thereafter. **(p. 382)**

Clinical Case 5

1. **The correct response is option B: Encourage the consumption of a diet that is low in fast food, sodas, and added sugar.**

   All pediatric patients should be encouraged to eat a balanced diet that consists of vegetables at most meals and avoiding foods that are high in fat, added salt, and sugar, such as fast food and soda (Table 26–2). Fruit drinks are another common source of hidden sugar, and their consumption should be limited. Obesity in the pediatric population is defined as a BMI greater than the 85th percentile, and lifestyle modifications should be initiated well before a patient meets this criterion. Aggressive interventions such as pharmacotherapy and a rigid dietary plan are not indicated for Sophia at this time. **(pp. 381, 383)**

2. **The correct response is option A: Group activities and team-based sports are encouraged above solitary activities.**

   All children and adolescents should be encouraged to exercise daily. Even when this goal is met, however, sedentary activities such as watching television and other forms of "screen time" should also be limited. Group activities such as team-based sports should be encouraged whenever they are available (see Table 26–2). **(p. 383)**

3. **The correct response is option D: BMI in the 90th percentile for age and sex.**

   Obesity in the pediatric population is defined as a BMI at or above the 85th percentile for the patient's age and sex, and warrants the urgent attention of the patient's primary care provider to assist in the development of an individualized plan for lifestyle modification. Regardless of the BMI percentile, a weight gain of greater than 7% attributed to an SGA should also secure immediate intervention. **(p. 381)**

TABLE 26–2. General diet and exercise plans for all child and adolescent patients

Diet

Patients should be encouraged to avoid drinking sodas and to limit intake of fruit drinks that are high in sugar.

Patients should be discouraged from eating fast food that may be high in fat, calories, or salt.

A balanced diet should include vegetables at most meals.

Patients should limit their intake of sugar.

Patients' weight should be monitored at each doctor visit, and patients should make dietary changes well before the body mass index reaches the 85th percentile.

The safest and most effective way to lose weight is to decrease caloric intake, per direction of a primary care provider. Medications such as metformin and topiramate are less effective, often have side effects, and should only rarely be used in treatment-refractory cases.

Exercise

All patients should be encouraged to exercise on a daily basis.

Sedentary activities outside of school should be limited (e.g., watching TV, using the computer, playing video games).

When available, group activities or team-based sports should be encouraged.

Clinical Case 6

1. **The correct response is option D: Decrease in overall calorie intake.**

   With the exception of insulin, all of the above would be expected to promote weight loss for this patient. However, decreasing calorie intake has been shown to be the safest and most effective way to lose weight, including the weight gain associated with the use of SGAs. It thus forms the foundation of the treatment plan for all obese youths. **(p. 383)**

2. **The correct response is option B: Topiramate.**

   No medications have U.S. Food and Drug Administration approval for the treatment of weight gain associated with SGA use, and none should be used routinely for this indication. However, the results of several trials suggest that metformin and topiramate are useful options for patients who are severely affected by SGA-facilitated weight gain when lifestyle modifications alone have been insufficient. **(pp. 381, 383)**

3. **The correct response is option A: Abdominal cramping.**

   Common side effects of metformin are diarrhea and abdominal cramping. Topiramate is commonly associated with cognitive dulling, paresthesias, dysesthesias, appetite suppression, and nephrolithiasis. **(p. 384)**

Clinical Case 7

1. **The correct response is option C: Approximately half of childhood-onset psychiatric disorders can be linked to childhood adversity.**

   Prior adversity is one of the strongest risk factors for future problems, and the effect is cumulative, with a greater number of experienced adversities correlating with increasing incidence of psychiatric disorders, including mood, anxiety, substance use, and disruptive behavior disorders. Childhood adversities, including sexual and physical abuse, have been associated with nearly half of all childhood-onset psychiatric disorders. There are similar correlations with adult-onset psychiatric disorders. **(p. 384)**

2. **The correct response is option D: Systematically screen for multiple potential types of childhood adversity and for symptoms associated with those events.**

   Children and adolescents should be screened for a variety of potential abuses and other types of adversity in a systematic fashion. Numerous validated instruments exist to assist clinicians in this endeavor. **(p. 385)**

3. **The correct response is option C: They tend to measure outcomes based on subsequent rates of abuse.**

   Child abuse prevention programs generally target families with younger children. They can be delivered in a variety of settings, typically in the home, in the primary care setting, or as part of other parent training programs. Outcome measurement tends to be based on subsequent rates of recidivism or abuse. **(p. 384)**

Clinical Case 8

1. **The correct response is option A: At every visit.**

   Suicide is a common cause of death among the pediatric population, particularly those with psychiatric disorders. Every child and adolescent should be screened for suicidal ideation at every mental health visit, with more intensive screening performed among those with significant risk factors. **(p. 385)**

2. **The correct response is option C: Peer who committed suicide.**

   By and large, suicide risk factors in children and adolescents mirror those in adults (Table 26–3). A notable exception is that children and adolescents are particularly susceptible to the contagion effect, having a significant increase in their risk of death by suicide after exposure to or knowledge of a peer or classmate who committed suicide. Suicide risk in the pediatric population is also particularly increased in the presence of family conflict. **(pp. 385–386)**

TABLE 26–3. **Risk factors for suicide in children and adolescents**
Previous history of suicide attempts
Recent exposure to a suicide or suicide attempt
High levels of anxiety
Hopelessness
History of substance misuse
Access to a gun
Command hallucinations
Contagion (i.e., having exposure to or knowledge of a suicide by a peer, classmate, etc.)
Physical or sexual abuse

3. **The correct response is option A: Major depressive disorder.**

   The risk of treatment-emergent suicidality should be discussed with the patient and parents before starting an antidepressant in a child or adolescent, and all such patients should be monitored carefully. However, one study suggested that the phenomenon is more prevalent among patients treated for a depressive disorder than among those treated for an anxiety disorder. **(p. 385)**

Clinical Case 9

1. **The correct response is option E: History of behavioral problems.**

   Risk factors for substance abuse among children and adolescents include male sex, a diagnosis of ADHD, and prior behavioral difficulties. **(p. 386)**

2. **The correct response is option C: Have you ever felt you needed to CUT down on your alcohol or drug use?**

   The questions included in the CRAFFT questionnaire for substance abuse screening in pediatric populations are listed in Table 26–4. The question in option C is a part of the CAGE instrument for alcohol misuse, which is commonly used in adults. **(p. 387)**

TABLE 26–4. The CRAFFT questionnaire for screening adolescents for substance abuse or misuse

C—Have you ever ridden in a CAR driven by someone (including yourself) who was "high" or had been using alcohol or drugs?
R—Do you ever use alcohol or drugs to RELAX, feel better about yourself, or fit in?
A—Do you ever use alcohol or drugs while you are ALONE?
F—Do your family or FRIENDS ever tell you that you should cut down on drinking or drug use?
F—Do you ever FORGET things you did while using alcohol or drugs?
T—Have you ever gotten into TROUBLE while you were using alcohol or drugs?

One positive answer suggests a need for more evaluation, while more than two affirmative responses suggest a significant problem.

Source. Knight JR, Sherritt L, Shrier LA, et al.: "Validity of the CRAFFT Substance Abuse Screening Test Among Adolescent Clinic Patients." *Archives of Pediatric and Adolescent Medicine* 156:607–614, 2002.

3. **The correct response is option D: Two or more positive responses suggest a significant substance use problem.**

   The CRAFFT questionnaire is a screening tool to identify adolescents (and young adults up to age 21) who are at high risk for substance use disorders and warrant further investigation into their substance use. It cannot be used to diagnose a substance use disorder, but a single positive response suggests a need for further evaluation, whereas two or more affirmative responses hint at a significant substance use problem. **(pp. 386–387)**

Clinical Case 10

1. **The correct response is option C: Two influenza vaccines are available for pediatric patients: the trivalent inactivated influenza vaccine and the live attenuated influenza vaccine.**

   Currently, immunization against influenza is recommended for all children older than 6 months. The live attenuated influenza vaccine is an alternative to the trivalent inactivated influenza vaccine for healthy children who do not have a severe chronic medical condition such as heart disease or a compromised immune system. Immunization recommendations in the United States are frequently updated by the Centers for Disease Control and Prevention (CDC). Physicians should consult the current vaccination schedule published annually by the CDC for the most up-to-date guidelines. Although many parents and guardians experience anxiety about perceived risks from vaccines, anticipatory guidance by physicians can markedly reduce their fears. **(pp. 386–388)**

2. **The correct response is option D: Immunoprophylaxis against human papillomavirus (HPV) is recommended to reduce the incidence of genital warts.**

   The HPV vaccine is currently approved for females ages 9–26 years to receive once, and is targeted to reduce the incidence of genital warts and abnormal cervical cytology, including cervical cancer. Immunization against *Neisseria meningitidis* is recommended to reduce the risk of meningitis. Adolescents should receive immunization with either the MCV4 vaccine or the MPSV4 vaccine between ages 11 and 12, with a booster dose at age 16. Both vaccines confer immunity against the same four serotypes of the *Neisseria meningitidis* bacterium. **(p. 387)**

Clinical Case 11

1. **The correct response is option D: Accidental injury.**

   Unintentional injuries, such as motor vehicle accidents, suffocation, poisonings, and gun violence, are the leading cause of death for children and adolescents. Therefore, screening for seat belt use is encouraged at every well-child visit. Patients should be advised to wear seat belts during every car trip. **(p. 388)**

2. **The correct response is option C: 60%.**

   Safety seats are recommended for young children and reduce the risk of fatality in a motor vehicle accident by 50%–70%. In addition, the current recommendations are that children should be seated in the back seat away from the airbag until they are older than age 13 years. **(p. 388)**

3. **The correct response is option A: Suffocation.**

   Suffocation is the leading cause of mortality in infants. Choking-related injuries are most often caused by coins, food, and toys. Small objects should be kept out of the environment of small children to prevent suffocation. **(p. 388)**

CHAPTER 27

Pain Medicine

Clinical Case 1

1. **The correct response is option A: Physical dependence.**

   Dependence is a state of adaptation that is manifested by a withdrawal syndrome that can be triggered by abrupt cessation, rapid dose reduction, or decreasing blood level of the drug, or administration of an antagonist. *Tolerance* is decreased duration of analgesia followed by decreased effectiveness. *Addiction* is compulsive use of a drug, preoccupation with the drug and its supply, inability to consistently control quantity used, craving of the psychological effects of the drug or urge to use the drug, and continued use despite adverse effects. *Abuse* may also indicate the habitual use of illegal drugs or the misuse of prescription or over-the-counter drugs with negative consequences that may include problems at work, in school, with interpersonal relationships, or with the law. **(pp. 403–404)**

2. **The correct response is option C: Review the Prescription Drug Monitoring Program (PDMP) database.**

   Accessing the PDMP database may indicate whether the patient is obtaining opioids from other physicians or emergency departments. At this point in time, it is not clear whether the patient has truly lost her medication more than once. It would not be prudent to write a prescription for opioids if the patient is consuming more medication than prescribed or misusing or diverting the medication, which may be considered aberrant behaviors. The patient requires counseling on medication safety and usage. It is not clear if the patient is doctor shopping or if she truly lost her medications. Discharging the patient without further investigation is not reasonable. **(pp. 401–402)**

3. **The correct response is option C: Check a urine drug screen.**

   The patient is exhibiting signs of acute methamphetamine use, which include pupil dilation, elevated blood pressure, and diaphoresis. Long-term use of methamphetamines may cause hypertension and heart attacks. An electrocardiogram would not address the patient's current state because she is not having chest pain or shortness of breath. A computed tomography (CT) scan would not be helpful because there is nothing to point toward intracranial pathology, and there are no signs of stroke. A urine drug screen would be helpful in determining which drugs the patient is using and guiding the clinician toward the next step in treatment. The patient is currently not complaining of symptoms suggestive of a myocardial infarction (e.g., fatigue; shortness of breath; chest, jaw, or back pain); therefore, checking cardiac enzymes are not indicated at this time. The patient is not likely experiencing a pulmonary embolism; these symptoms would include shortness of breath, sharp sudden chest pain, rapid heart rate, anxiety, and coughing up pink frothy mucus. **(p. 402)**

Clinical Case 2

1. **The correct response is option B: "I was an alcoholic for 12 years."**

   The acronym AMPS stands for **A**nxiety, **M**ood, **P**sychosis, and **S**ubstance abuse (Figure 27–1), and therefore is useful for assessing Ms. Wilson's alcoholism. The statements about snoring and gasping for air suggest an obstructive process occurring during sleep; this information would be elicited using the STOP-BANG Questionnaire to screen for obstructive sleep apnea (see Figure 27–4 later in this chapter). The rating of pain severity is information obtained from the PQRST tool for the assessment of pain symptoms. PQRST stands for **P**rovoking events, **Q**uality of symptoms, **R**egion and radiation of symptoms, **S**everity, and **T**ime frame. The statement about running out of opioid medication and asking for early refills shows aberrant behavior. The assessment of opioid management can be determined with the 4 A's (**A**nalgesia, **A**ctivities, **A**dverse reactions, **A**berrancy) (see Figure 27–3 later in this chapter). This aberrant behavior is also represented as the S (substance use) on the AMPS assessment of psychiatric illness, but this tool is geared toward a brief psychiatric and illicit substance use screen. **(pp. 394–399, 405)**

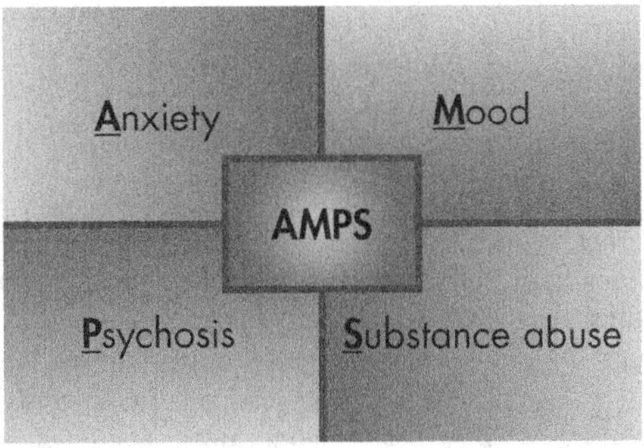

FIGURE 27–1. AMPS psychiatric assessment.

Source. Adapted from McCarron RM, Xiong GL, Bourgeois J: *Lippincott's Primary Care Psychiatry: For Primary Care Clinicians and Trainees, Medical Specialists, Neurologists, Emergency Medical Professionals, Mental Health Providers, and Trainees.* Philadelphia, PA, Lippincott Williams & Wilkins, 2009.

2. **The correct response is option E: Try treatment with a topical anesthetic.**

   The first step of the three-step analgesic ladder (Figure 27–2), which is for mild to moderate pain rated as 5 or below on the visual analog scale, is to try treatment with nonopioid medications (acetaminophen, NSAIDs, gabapentinoids, antidepressants, anticonvulsants, or topical agents). Before a medication is dismissed as a failure, the patient should take the appropriate dose on a scheduled interval for at least 2 weeks, barring significant side effects. If the nonopioid trial has been unsuccessful and pain persists without functional improvement, movement to the second step is warranted. **(p. 404)**

3. **The correct response is option E: Answers B and D.**

   Urine drug screens and PDMP database searches are useful tools if you suspect illicit drug use and to guide in adherence monitoring. Each step of the three-step analgesic ladder should include history and physical examination, 2- to 4-week minimal duration trial of medications, interventional pain procedures if indicated, lifestyle modifications, and a plan to reassess pain and functionality (see Figure 27–2). **(p. 404)**

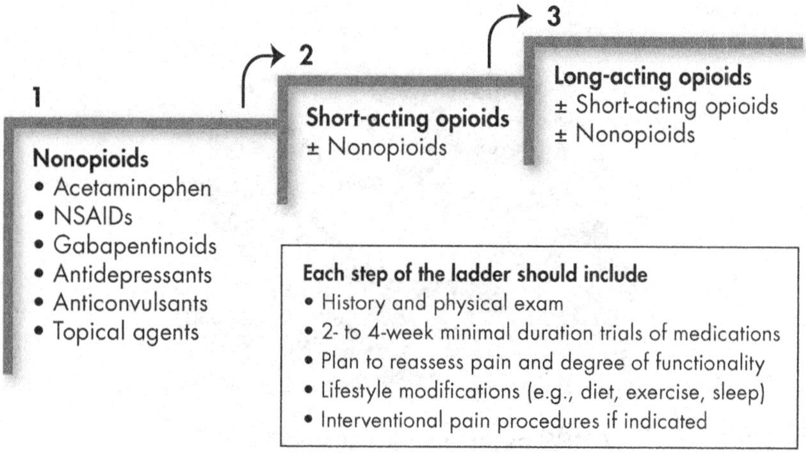

FIGURE 27–2. Three-step analgesic ladder.

NSAID = nonsteroidal anti-inflammatory drug.

Source. Adapted from World Health Organization: *Cancer Pain Relief: With a Guide to Opioid Availability,* 2nd Edition. Geneva, Switzerland, World Health Organization, 1996.

4. **The correct response is option A: Neck circumference of 36 cm.**

   The STOP-BANG Questionnaire is a tool used to assess obstructive sleep apnea risk (see Figure 27–4 later in this chapter). The tool includes eight factors that are used for risk stratification. The presence of three or more of the following categorizes the patient as high risk: loud snoring, daytime tiredness, observed apnea, hypertension, BMI greater than 35, age over 50 years, neck girth above 40 cm for men or above 35 cm for women, and male gender. **(p. 398)**

Clinical Case 3

1. **The correct response is option E: Answers B and D.**

   Random urine drug screens and PDMP database searches are used to guide a clinician in adherence monitoring and to look for drug misuse. A CD4 count is a useful test for following the integrity of the immune system and is indicative of the HIV disease stage. Liver function tests are likely not needed at this point. Both tests gather important information but will not change the patient's immediate state of health and treatment. **(pp. 402–403)**

2. **The correct response is option E: Neuropathic pain.**

   Two general classes of pain are neuropathic and nociceptive pain. Neuropathic pain is characteristically described as tingling, numbness, "pins and needles," shooting, or electric-like and results from ongoing nerve stimulation or abnormal messaging in the peripheral and central nervous system. Nociceptive pain is divided into somatic and visceral pain. Nociceptive pain is caused by primary afferent nerve injury or peripheral inflammation. Somatic pain is described using descriptors such as *dull, aching, pressure,* and *sharp.* Visceral pain is usually poorly localized. Referred somatic pain is when pathology in one area causes pain in another area. **(pp. 395–396)**

3. **The correct response is option E: All of the above.**

   The patient is taking a large dose of opioids and is at risk for developing tolerance. He has been taking larger doses of opioids over the past 4 years, presumably due to decreased effectiveness or shortened effect. Other common side effects of opioids include sedation, respiratory depression, impaired judgment, impaired coordination, constipation, nausea, accelerated loss of bone mineral density, and opioid-induced hyperalgesia. Hyperalgesia is a syndrome that includes increased sensitivity to painful stimuli, worsening pain despite increasing doses of opioids, and pain that extends beyond the distribution of existing pain. Accidental death is the most serious possible result. The risk of opioid-related accidental death is significantly increased when opioids are used concomitantly with other medications, such as benzodiazepines, that have concomitant side effects of sedation and respiratory impairment. **(pp. 403–404)**

Clinical Case 4

1. **The correct response is option C: Adequate pain relief and increased daily activity.**

   The 4 A's assessment method is used for monitoring outcomes for patients on opioid therapy (Figure 27–3). Although tobacco use is associated with increased pain, it is not assessed using the 4 A's. The patient drinks alcohol in amounts that are not considered in excess of normal use. If the patient were to use alcohol and opioids at the same time, this would be a demonstration of aberrant behavior. Poor compliance with continuous positive airway pressure (CPAP) is important information and may adversely affect the patient's health. If the patient continues to fail to use her CPAP machine, the physician may need to have a conversation with the patient regarding continuation of opioid therapy. **(p. 405)**

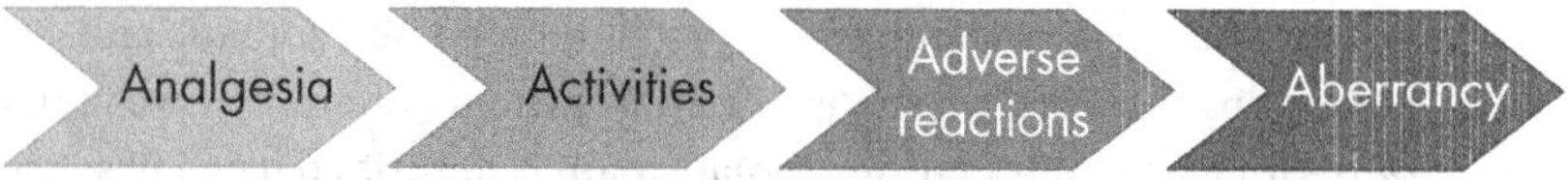

FIGURE 27–3. Assessment of opioid management with the "4 A's."
The 4 A's is a simple method to monitor outcomes once a patient begins opioid therapy. These factors should be assessed at every office visit to help guide ongoing treatment.

2. **The correct response is option B: Depression.**

The AMPS psychiatric assessment is used to look for potential psychiatric pain generators (see Figure 27–1). The patient describes sleep disturbances, loss of energy, and loss of interest (anhedonia) in previously enjoyable activities. These are all signs of depression that can make the patient's pain worse. **(pp. 397–398)**

3. **The correct response is option E: All of the above.**

The clinician should avoid passing judgment when aberrant behavior is demonstrated but should also be vigilant in assessing a patient's behavior. Respectful scrutiny is warranted because the patient may be taking more of the medication than is prescribed, which can be life threatening (misuse or abuse), or giving the medication to a friend or family member (diversion). Prescription opioids are currently a drug of abuse and have a high street value. It is the prescribing provider's responsibility to determine how the opioids are being used. Because the PDMP database shows that Ms. Aterman has visited several providers for opioid prescriptions and has made several visits to the emergency department for opioids, she is stratified as being at high risk of opioid use disorder. **(pp. 402–403)**

4. **The correct response is option C: Urine drug screens every 3–6 months.**

   Once a patient's risk is stratified as being low, moderate, or high, adherence monitoring can be determined. Low-risk patients should have urine drug screening every 6–12 months and have the PDMP reviewed at drug initiation and three times per year. High-risk patients should have urine drug screening every 3–6 months and have the PDMP reviewed at drug initiation and four or more times per year. **(p. 403)**

Clinical Case 5

1. **The correct response is option C: Untreated anxiety.**

   Posttraumatic stress disorder is a type of anxiety condition primarily marked by a reexperiencing of the traumatic event (e.g., through flashbacks or dreams of the trauma) and by a hyperarousal or hyperstartle response, which may increase muscle tension and subsequently worsen the pain. Poor blood glucose control over time has been shown to cause nonenzymatic glycosylation of peripheral nerves, resulting in neuropathic pain. However, Ms. Davis is not describing neuropathic pain. Poor compliance with medical care can be problematic and make ongoing care difficult. Not following medical directions for medications or recommended adjunct treatment modalities will likely not escalate pain. Alcohol abuse can amplify a patient's pain level; however, occasional nonexcessive use of alcohol has not been shown to cause escalation of baseline pain levels. **(p. 398)**

2. **The correct response is option A: No further actions.**

   In accordance with the World Health Organization's three-step analgesic ladder, treatment should begin with a nonopioid medication. A medication trial is not a failure until the patient has taken an appropriate dose at a scheduled interval for at least 2 weeks. The first step also includes adding adjuvant treatments, which may include anticonvulsants, antidepressants, topical agents, anxiolytics, antipsychotics, and muscle relaxants. Ms. Davis has been taking an antidepressant and an NSAID for several months, but this treatment has failed. The next step is to start a short-acting opioid with an endpoint in mind. It is not necessary to trial another NSAID prior to the next step because the patient has failed therapy with an NSAID and an antidepressant for an appropriate length of time. **(pp. 403–404)**

3. **The correct response is option C: Tolerance.**

Tolerance is the body's ability to become adjusted to a substance so that its effects are less strong than previously experienced with the same amount. Dependence is a state of adaptation in which an organism functions normally only in the presence of that substance. Addiction is the compulsive need for and use of a substance characterized by tolerance and by physiological symptoms upon withdrawal of that substance. Abuse is the patterned use of a substance in which the individual uses the substance in amounts that are harmful to themselves or others. Drug diversion involves the use or selling of medications for recreational purposes. **(pp. 403–404)**

4. **The correct response is option D: Accidental death.**

The risk of opioid-related accidental death is significantly increased when opioids are mixed with benzodiazepines. Opioids interfere with the hypothalamic-pituitary-gonadal axis, causing reductions of adrenal androgen production; the addition of benzodiazepines would not contribute to the suppression of the sex steroids. Hyperalgesia is a syndrome of increased sensitivity to painful stimuli, worsening pain despite increasing doses of opioids, and pain that extends beyond the distribution of existing pain. Although Ms. Davis may have hyperalgesia, this syndrome is unrelated to the addition of a benzodiazepine. A patient who has been taking opioids for an extended period of time is at risk for developing tolerance. Ms. Davis has been taking escalating doses of opioids over the past 14 months, presumably because of decreased effectiveness or duration of effect. The addition of benzodiazepines does not affect tolerance. Patients who have been using opioids for a long time are at higher risk of developing bone loss and osteoporosis. The exact mechanism is unknown but appears to be multifactorial. Contributing factors include the development of an endocrinopathy, direct osteoblast inhibition, and the effects of associated comorbidities. **(p. 404)**

Clinical Case 6

1. **The correct response is option B: Thyroid-stimulating hormone test.**

Hypothyroidism can lead to fatigue, whole body aches, weight gain, poor motivation, poor concentration, depression, and generalized myofascial pain. Thyroid irregularities can be easily investigated with blood tests, and Ms. Bradford's symptoms are most indicative of low thyroid hormone. Poorly controlled blood pressure and blood glucose can worsen headaches and lead to peripheral neuropathy. Pseudotumor cerebri, detected using head and neck CT scan, can occur in obese women and cause headaches, but can also cause neck/shoulder pain, blurred vision, and tinnitus; Ms. Bradford does not exhibit most of these symptoms, making the diagnosis less likely. A complete blood count can detect infection, inflammation, anemia, and a wide variety of disorders. Obesity increases the risk of developing fatty liver disease and other diseases that can elevate liver enzymes. Although elevated liver enzymes can cause headaches, they do not cause the constellation of symptoms described in the case description. **(p. 394)**

2. **The correct response is option E: Answers A, B, and C.**

   The STOP-BANG Questionnaire is used to screen for obstructive sleep apnea (Figure 27–4). Patients with three or more "yes" answers have a high risk for sleep apnea and should be evaluated further by a sleep specialist. Ms. Bradford meets several high-risk findings that point toward an obstructive sleep apnea diagnosis: loud snoring (often heard through closed doors), a calculated BMI of 37.8, and daytime tiredness. Being male but not female is considered a positive finding for obstructive sleep apnea on the STOP-BANG Questionnaire. **(p. 398)**

3. **The correct response is option D: Trigger point injections.**

   A true trigger point is described as a focal spot within a taught muscle band that causes a radiating referral pattern or motor or autonomic dysfunction. Treatments that have been shown to be beneficial for trigger points include physical therapy, massage, ultrasound, dry needling, and injection with local anesthetic, botulinum toxin, or corticosteroid. Patients with axial back pain that radiates to the posterior thigh can have facet-mediated pain that may benefit from a radiofrequency ablation of the medial branch nerves. Patients with radicular spine pain have nerve root impingement; their pain is frequently described as electrical, burning, or shooting in behavior. These patients may benefit from an epidural steroid injection. Facet-mediated pain in the cervical or lumbar region can be relieved with steroid injections near the joint. The physical examination in Ms. Bradford's case does not point toward facet-mediated pain. **(pp. 405–406)**

SNORE: Do you snore loudly enough to be heard through closed doors?	Yes/No
TIRED: Do you often feel tired, without energy, and sleepy during the day?	Yes/No
OBSERVED: Have you been observed to stop breathing while you were sleeping?	Yes/No
PRESSURE: Do you have or are you being treated for high blood pressure?	Yes/No
BODY MASS INDEX (BMI): What is your BMI? Is it >35?	Yes/No
AGE: Is your age over 50 years old?	Yes/No
NECK GIRTH: Do you have a neck circumference >40 cm (male), >35 cm (female)?	Yes/No
GENDER: Are you a male?	Yes/No

FIGURE 27–4. STOP-BANG Questionnaire: a tool to screen for obstructive sleep apnea (OSA) risk.

Note. High risk of OSA with ≥3 answers of "yes." Additional workup by a sleep specialist or by polysomnography is indicated.
Low risk of OSA with <3 answers of "yes."
Source. Adapted from STOP Questionnaire (Chung F, Elsaid H: "Screening for Obstructive Sleep Apnea Before Surgery: Why Is It Important?" *Current Opinion in Anesthesiology* 22(3):405–411, 2009).

Clinical Case 7

1. **The correct response is option C: Obstructive sleep apnea.**

   Obstructive and central types of sleep apnea are common causes of sleep disturbances and should be thoroughly evaluated prior to prescribing an opiate or other potentially sedating medication. Undiagnosed sleep apnea combined with opioids and/or benzodiazepines leads to increased morbidity and mortality. Coronary artery disease, diabetes, and hyperlipidemia are serious medical conditions but do not necessarily need to be ruled out before a patient starts taking an opiate. **(pp. 397, 408)**

2. **The correct response is option B: STOP-BANG.**

   The acronym STOP-BANG stands for the eight components of a rapid screen for obstructive sleep apnea (see Figure 27–4). Three or more "yes" responses represent a high risk of obstructive sleep apnea. A-SCAR is a mnemonic that helps in remembering the treatment of obesity among individuals with serious mental illness (**A**ssess, **S**witch, **C**hange, **A**dd, **R**efer). VITAMIN D is a mnemonic frequently used to evaluate the etiology for different pathological processes (**V**ascular, **I**nfectious, **T**rauma, **A**utoimmune, **M**etabolic, **I**nherited, **N**eoplastic, **D**rug). CREATE is a mnemonic that helps providers create cultural competence (**C**ollaborate, **R**eflect, **E**mpathize, **A**ncillary, **T**iming, **E**ducate). **(p. 398)**

3. **The correct response is option C: Referral for a sleep study.**

   Mr. Sidel scores 5 on STOP-BANG (tired, pressure, BMI>35, age>50, male gender) (see Figure 27–4). Anyone scoring 3 or more is considered to be at high risk for obstructive sleep apnea, and additional workup by a sleep specialist or by polysomnography is indicated. This additional workup should take place before a trial of an opiate medication. Consideration could be given to a retrial of gabapentin at a lower dose; however, workup for obstructive sleep apnea should take priority. Tramadol is an opiate-like medication and carries many of the same risks as traditional opiates, including respiratory depression. **(p. 398)**

Clinical Case 8

1. **The correct response is option A: Anxiety.**

   AMPS is an acronym for **A**nxiety, **M**ood, **P**sychosis, and **S**ubstance abuse (see Figure 27–1). Mr. Vincent exhibits anxious symptoms and has a clinical presentation that likely meets the criteria for somatic symptom disorder, with predominant pain. The patient may also have a mood disorder, but anxiety is the main psychiatric pain generator. **(pp. 398–399)**

2. **The correct response is option D: Cognitive-behavioral therapy.**

   Cognitive-behavioral therapy is the first-line treatment choice to reduce the anxious symptoms associated with this kind of somatic symptom disorder. Pharmacotherapy with a selective serotonin reuptake inhibitor is also efficacious. Physical therapy, acupuncture, and meditation are potential adjunctive treatment modalities. **(pp. 394, 405)**

3. **The correct response is option E: Answers A and B.**

   Untreated anxiety can be a tremendous amplifier of any pain condition. Anxiety propagates a vicious cycle of intensified sympathetic response that, if left untreated, will maintain the pain. Anxious rumination can impair sleep, which can in turn impair function and lead to worsened pain. Anxiety is not usually associated with an increase in malingered symptoms. A good doctor-patient relationship can decrease anxiety symptoms. **(p. 398)**

Clinical Case 9

1. **The correct response is option D: Myofascial pain syndrome.**

   The patient describes classic trigger points consistent with myofascial pain syndrome. Disc herniation with radicular pain would most likely present with pain radiating down the leg. Patients with facet arthropathy often present with axial lower back pain that may or may not radiate as far distally as the posterior thigh. Fibromyalgia typically consists of widespread musculoskeletal pain and fatigue, with tender points in multiple locations. **(pp. 405–406)**

2. **The correct response is option B: Trigger point injection.**

   Myofascial pain syndrome may be treated with trigger point needle injections with local anesthetic, corticosteroid, or botulinum toxin, or with dry needling. Facet arthropathy is treated with radiofrequency ablation of the medial branch nerves innervating arthritic facet joints. Epidural steroid injections are used for radicular spine pain such as that found following lumbar disc herniation. Complex regional pain syndrome can be treated with a sympathetic block. **(pp. 405–406)**

3. **The correct response is option A: Hyperirritable spot with referred symptoms.**

   Hyperirritable spots with referred symptoms are called trigger points. Multiple points of tenderness throughout the body are typical for fibromyalgia; these tender points do not have referred symptoms, although palpation of trigger points creates pain in areas other than the location of the trigger point itself. Radicular spine pain is typically not associated with a taut muscle band or hyperirritable spot. The referred symptoms associated with a trigger point can include motor or autonomic dysfunction, but these symptoms are not required for the diagnosis. **(pp. 405–406)**

Clinical Case 10

1. **The correct response is option C: Diabetic peripheral neuropathy.**

   Diabetic peripheral neuropathy classically presents with paresthesia in a stocking and glove distribution as described in this case. Spondylolisthesis (displacement of one vertebra over another) can cause bilateral leg pain and paresthesia, but the pain typically presents as radiating pain starting in the back and radiating down one or both legs. Degenerative disc disease can result in lower extremity neuropathic pain if there is encroachment on a spinal nerve; however, this would typically present as radiating back pain down one leg. The pain from fibromyalgia is typically whole body with multiple points of tenderness. **(pp. 395, 405–406)**

2. **The correct response is option A: Duloxetine.**

   The first-line treatment of neuropathic pain almost always involves the use of nonopioid medications, such as tricyclic antidepressants, anticonvulsants, and serotonin-norepinephrine reuptake inhibitors (SNRIs). Among the choices, duloxetine, amitriptyline, and gabapentin have shown benefit in treating neuropathic pain, and duloxetine and amitriptyline are indicated for treatment of depression. In a 67-year-old patient, duloxetine would likely be preferred over amitriptyline given its more favorable side-effect profile. **(p. 399)**

3. **The correct response is option C: By increasing appetite.**

   Mirtazapine is an efficacious antidepressant for the treatment of major depressive disorder. However, it is associated with increased appetite, which may present a problem for this patient with uncontrolled diabetes and obesity. It is not associated with an increased sensitivity to neuropathic pain, and it typically improves sleep. **(pp. 146, 399)**

Clinical Case 11

1. **The correct response is option B: Lumbar facet arthropathy.**

   Patients with lumbar facet arthropathy typically have axial lower back pain; there can be radiation as far distally as the posterior thigh but typically not below the knee. Disc herniation with impingement of a nerve root would classically involve radiating pain down the length of one leg. Spinal stenosis of the lumbar spine often involves numbness, paresthesia, or weakness in both lower extremities worsened by activity. Diabetic neuropathy usually manifests as bilateral paresthesia in a stocking and glove distribution. **(pp. 405–406)**

2. **The correct response is option A: Nonsteroidal anti-inflammatory drug (NSAID).**

   NSAIDs are recommended for inflammatory pain such as that found with lumbar facet arthropathy. Anticonvulsants and the SNRIs are recommended for neuropathic pain. Myofascial pain and fibromyalgia may also respond to the SNRIs. Opiates are reserved for those who are unsuccessful with a trial of nonopioid analgesics. **(pp. 399, 403)**

3. **The correct response is option D: Radiofrequency ablation.**

   Radiofrequency ablation of the medial branch nerves innervating arthritic facet joints may reduce axial back pain and associated referred pain. Epidural steroid injections may be beneficial for radicular spinal pain. Trigger point injections can be helpful in the treatment of myofascial pain syndrome. Transcutaneous electrical nerve stimulation (TENS) is not an interventional procedure. **(pp. 405–406)**

Clinical Case 12

1. **The correct response is option B: Oxycodone.**

   Opioids represent a significant risk in this patient with possible obstructive sleep apnea (she screens positive on the STOP-BANG Questionnaire for tired, hypertension, BMI, and age; see Figure 27–4 earlier in this chapter) and other related side effects including respiratory depression. Undiagnosed sleep apnea combined with opioids leads to increased morbidity and mortality. **(pp. 398, 405)**

2. **The correct response is option A: Weight loss guidance.**

   Overweight and obese patients should have nutritional assessment and weight loss guidance as part of their comprehensive pain treatment program. This patient has grade III obesity, and her obesity is likely the main contributor to her pain. It is unlikely that she would be able to participate in yoga. TENS and acupuncture could provide some relief. **(p. 405)**

3. **The correct response is option D: Obstructive sleep apnea and multiple sedating medications.**

   Ms. Schulte has four of the eight risk factors for obstructive sleep apnea on the STOP-BANG Questionnaire (see Figure 27–4). Nighttime hypoxia leads to frequent bouts of sleep arousal, which can lead to daytime somnolence. She is also taking multiple sedating medications, including gabapentin, OxyContin, oxycodone, and paroxetine. There is no evidence that the patient's sleep is interrupted by ruminating thoughts. Her pain is worse with ambulation than while sleeping. **(p. 397)**

CPSIA information can be obtained
at www.ICGtesting.com
Printed in the USA
FSOW04n0802271016
26584FS

9 781615 370573